Why Am I a Dentist?

Why Am I a Dentist?

A search for clarity and meaning

DR MAX LEE

First published in 2024 by Dean Publishing
PO Box 119
Mt. Macedon, Victoria, 3441
Australia
deanpublishing.com

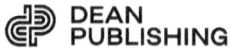

Copyright © Dr Max Lee

All rights reserved. No part of this publication may be reproduced, stored in a retrieval system or transmitted in any way or by any means, electronic, mechanical, photocopying, recording or otherwise, without the prior written permission of the publisher.

Cataloguing-in-Publication Data
National Library of Australia
Title: Why Am I a Dentist? — A Search for Clarity and Meaning
Edition: 1st edn
ISBN: 978-0-648758-01-3
Category: Dentistry

The views and opinions expressed in this book are those of the author and do not necessarily reflect the official policy or position of any other agency, publisher, organisation, employer, board, association or company. Assumptions made in the analysis are not reflective of the position of any entity other than the author(s) — and, these views are always subject to change, revision, and rethinking at any time. This book is only to be used as a source of thought, inspiration and humour and not to be used to diagnose dental or medical issues.

The author, publisher or organisations are not to be held responsible for misuse, reuse, recycled and cited and/or uncited copies of content within this book by others.

This book and its opinions reflect the author's ideas only and are not to be used without appropriate consultation with your own doctor or your own medical or dental professional. The reader should always consult a physician in matters relating to his/her health and particularly with respect to any symptoms that may require diagnosis or medical attention. The ideas within this book are not intended to replace any medical advice nor do they reflect any dental or medical body or organisation. The author's personal philosophy and story are mere narratives and accounts as remembered at the time. Some names and places may have been changed to protect the identity of certain people.

This book is dedicated to my patients over the years whose collective sacrifice has led to my levelling up as a dentist.

CONTENTS

Introduction ~ ix

Chapter 1
Student Days ~ 1

Chapter 2
Singapore Days,
Earlier ~ 9

Chapter 3
Singapore Days,
Latter ~ 15

Chapter 4
On Orthodontic
Treatments ~ 27

Chapter 5
On Patients ~ 35

Chapter 6
On Dental
Procedures ~ 55

Chapter 7
On the Dental
Industry ~ 79

Chapter 8
Money Matters ~ 103

Chapter 9
On Hamlet and
Doenjang-Jjigae ~ 121

Chapter 10
On Being a Dentist ~ 135

**Frequently Asked Questions, and
Brutally Honest Answers** ~ 142

About the Author ~ 145

Endnotes ~ 146

INTRODUCTION

Before I started writing this book, I did a quick online search and found that there has been no book, at least in the English-speaking world, that tells the stories of dentists and the dental industry. There are dental textbooks designed for dental students; there are picture books aimed at preparing toddlers for their first dental visit; there are compilations of dental jokes; there are guidance books for dental practice management, but no book that portrays the lives of dentists and the happenings of the dental world. One must wonder why. Other professional worlds such as medical, legal and financial have given birth to plenty of books, TV series, podcasts and other forms of media that tell the stories of those worlds. Medical dramas constantly rank among the most popular TV series on various streaming platforms. Why, then, is there such a scarcity of media in the market that tell the stories of dentists? In other words, why are dentists not writing about their own lives?

I can offer three explanations. First, a dentist may feel shy about sharing the various workplace happenings with the rest of the world. The majority of dramas that dentists experience throughout their careers are interpersonal conflicts with patients, other dentists and other staff members. These are unpleasant episodes that one is usually not too excited to share with people outside their immediate social circle. Second, a dentist may fear the legal repercussions of publishing sensitive content. If a dentist wrote about their patients or other dentists, those individuals may be offended for whatever reason and sue. Those lawsuits may or may not have legitimate grounds, but dentists are risk-averse creatures who like to avoid in the first place engaging in any activity that may potentially lead to legal trouble. Third, a dentist may feel uncomfortable about discussing the various norms and conventions of the dental industry, lest they be labelled a 'rebel' or a 'disruptor' by the dental community. Dentistry is an ancient profession, and ancient professions have norms and conventions that their members are expected to follow without question.

INTRODUCTION

I am not immune to the psychological forces mentioned that discourage dentists from writing about their own world. I, too, feel shy about publishing my episodes of interpersonal conflicts with my colleagues. I, too, feel nervous about publishing my opinions on the inner workings of the dental industry. I have faith, however, in the positive impacts that can be generated from writing about difficult topics, which is what emboldens me to share the memories that I am embarrassed to share, and address the topics that I am afraid to address. While I was working on this book, I shared bits and pieces of it with dentists around me, and some of the common responses were: "Thank you for deciding to share your experiences" and, "You are brave to write about these difficult topics." These kind words from my colleagues reveal to me something: dentists yearn for a book in the market that tells their story. Dentists, like anyone, seek to be understood, which is best achieved when one shares their worries and concerns with the rest of the world. It's just that no dentist has yet dared to pick up the mantle of storyteller, due to the various psychological impediments listed above. I volunteer to take up that mantle.

I graduated dental school in 2013. I have thought about writing a book on dentistry since new-graduate days, but thought it was best to wait until I had accumulated sufficient experience in the field. As a new-graduate dentist, I had things to say, but felt that more years in the trade would provide me the perspective I needed to be able to examine my own life and my own career from various angles. I have been a dentist for more than a decade now, and feel that I am able to 'zoom out' on my own life and career better than I used to.

I aim to achieve three things by writing this book. First, I want to share the various aspects of working as a dentist, in the hope of humanising this profession about which so little is known by the outside world. I know that the public typically perceives dentists as cold-blooded money-grubbers who wield a needle in one hand and a drill in the other – I hope to defuse that perception and show the world that there is a living, breathing person behind the dental mask. Second, I aim to address and comment on a range of issues surrounding the private dental industry, in the hope of sparking a discussion on the topics that dentists usually hesitate to talk about. I might rub a few people the wrong way in the process, but I am not scared. It is a risk that all authors have to take. A quick note here is that my commentary on private dentistry is based on Australian and Singaporean contexts – two countries where I have expe-

INTRODUCTION

rience practising. Third, I aim to answer a question that I have been asking myself since day one of my career, but have struggled to answer: *Why am I a dentist?* I know that many dentists ask themselves the same question every day. If you are like me and have an identity crisis every morning as you walk through the dental clinic, I believe you will find it worthwhile to join me on this journey as I seek to answer what the profession of dentistry means to me personally.

So, let us dive in.

WHY AM I A DENTIST?

CHAPTER 1

STUDENT DAYS

I finished high school in 2008. Australian dental schools in my day looked at two main criteria for entry: ENTER (Equivalent National Tertiary Entrance Rank) score and UMAT (Undergraduate Medicine Admission Test) score. In addition, some universities required applicants to attend in-person interviews. My ENTER score was 99.90, which was high enough to compensate for my relatively low UMAT score of 80. I applied to all dental schools in Australia and received offers from two of them: the University of Melbourne and the University of Adelaide. As a

Melbourne resident, my natural choice was the University of Melbourne.

I am ashamed to admit that I was never a keen student in dental school. I did not choose to study dentistry out of some noble sense of duty. My patients ask me all the time why I chose to study dentistry, and I always stutter because I never know what to say. The honest answer is that I was 19 at the time and had not reached the stage in life where one makes proactive career choices based on articulable reasons. My parents, teachers and friends all told me that going to dental school would be sensible, and I went along with their recommendations.

In dental school, I studied barely enough to scrape a pass for all my subjects. My reasoning at the time for being a slacker was this: whether I studied hard and got good grades or slacked off and just passed all my examinations, the end result would be the same – a dental licence that doesn't discriminate based on university grades – so why put in the extra effort? Why aim for a distinction when a pass is sufficient? Far better, I told my silly self, to divert free time elsewhere for self-development in areas other than dentistry. I proudly slacked off. I partied and socialised. I walked past the university library sometimes and shook my head at other dental students who tucked themselves into the library without having even a bit of a social life. Looking back, I think it was a silly attitude for me to have.

People say that dentistry must have been difficult to study. Since I have only completed one tertiary degree in my life, I cannot comment whether dentistry is more difficult than other degrees or courses. We dentists certainly like to claim so because it supports the narrative that dentists deserve a high pay. I am sure that all university studies come with their own sets of challenges and are all difficult in their own unique ways. Studying dentistry was, of course, not a walk in the park. Every exam period was a struggle. Every year, at least one or two students from the cohort failed one of the end-of-year examinations, forcing them to stay back a year. I would say that a reasonably intelligent person with a reasonable level of self-discipline can make it through dental school. Look at me, I am neither super intelligent nor super disciplined, but I've made it.

The parties and the social activities that I indulged in during the first few years of university paid off. I was elected as the president of Melbourne Dental Students' Society (MDSS) in my fourth year of studies. Bachelor of Dental Science is a 5-year degree, but it was customary at Melbourne Dental School for fourth-year students to take leadership roles because final year students were too busy with their studies.

The traditional role of MDSS was to organise and host all the social activities, including orientation programs for new students, annual student camp, and the annual student ball. But I wanted MDSS to be more than just an organiser of parties. I looked for ways to improve the welfare of fellow dental students, whose interests I represented. An issue soon caught my attention. In dental school, there were practical sessions where students practised various types of dental procedures on mannequin heads, fitted with plastic tooth models. The tooth models could only be practised on once before being discarded. Students could purchase new tooth models from the school office for $4 per piece. Since students, including myself, made heaps of mistakes during the practical sessions, it was not uncommon for students to burn through $20-30 per session, which was not an insignificant sum for students. Remember, this was back in the 2010s when one could get a takeaway meal and a drink for less than $10. After some research, I found out that I could order the same brand of plastic tooth models in bulk, directly from the supplier, at a unit price lower than what the dental school charged. The student committee would then be able to sell them to dental students for about

$2 per piece, since we did not have to make any profit from them. I did not see any problem with it. It was an initiative that would benefit all dental students, and in my view the kind of initiative that a student committee should pursue. Unfortunately, other members of the committee did not see it that way. At a meeting, I gave the pitch to my committee, and the response was lukewarm. The committee members looked at me as though I was going above and beyond to look for unnecessary trouble. So I gave up my plans. It was my first little lesson that, in politics, impetus is often met with inertia. To be fair to my committee, organising and hosting all the social activities took a considerable amount of time and effort, so I cannot blame them for not wanting to do more than what they were conventionally expected to do.

The committee met almost every day to discuss and organise upcoming events. The biggest event of the MDSS calendar was the annual dental ball, which took forever to organise. The Grand Dental Ball of 2012, I can confidently say, was the best dental ball in the history of Melbourne Dental School. For two reasons. One, according to ancient Mayan legend, 2012 was supposed to be the year the world ended. A movie was even made about it. So we all danced at the ball like there was no tomorrow. Second, around the time of the dental ball, Gangnam Style by PSY was at the peak of its global craze. So, at the ball, we all danced to the tune of Gangnam Style. Beat that.

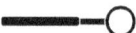

I burnt out by the end of the year, not from all the organisation tasks – for I loved doing them – but from all the socialising that was part and parcel of being on the student committee. I almost developed a quasi social phobia. I had met so many new people and made so much small talk as president that, by the end of my tenure, I was scared of bumping into people at university, making small talk or even saying hi to people I recognised. I got scared of using the elevator in the dental school building because, when the elevator stopped and the door opened, someone I knew might come onto the elevator, and I would have to make small talk with them until the elevator reached my level. I almost contemplated wearing a face covering around the dental school so people would not recognise me, but quickly abandoned the idea because I would be the only person in the building to wear a face covering, which would make me even more conspicuous. In the dental school building, I often walked briskly past people I knew, pretending not to recognise them. I must have looked so arrogant. It is one of the things I regret.

All that is not to say that I did not enjoy my time as president. It was such a rewarding experience, and to serve the needs of my fellow students for a year was a great personal honour. I was immensely proud that I represented the students of the best dental school in Australia. I wish all current and future MDSS presidents a successful tenure, and would like to remind them that if they need any advice, I am just a Facebook message away.

Fifth and final year of dental school was tough. I coped with the stress of studying for the final examinations by eating through a pack of Tim Tams a day for 3 consecutive months. I gained almost 10 kg in 3 months. I failed one of the examinations and had to resit it but passed the second time. All those Tim Tams had done their magic! I would like to reassure all dental students reading this that failing an examination is okay; it can happen to anyone, and unless you are really, really bad, the professors will usually try to pass you the second time.

WHY AM I A DENTIST?

CHAPTER 2

SINGAPORE DAYS, EARLIER

Final year dental students had to deal with the additional stress of looking for their first employment after graduation. As the final examinations approached, tensions grew between final-year students regarding job positions that were available for new graduates. Like any other industry, few dental practices are willing to hire new graduates. Job positions that accept applications from new graduates are slim pickings. So, in my final year, when students found a job advertisement that did not include that dreaded phrase, 'experienced dentists only', they kept the information to themselves, hoping that no one else would apply for the same position. This led to some hilarious situations. A student might find a job opening at some interstate dental clinic, book a flight for the job interview without telling anyone, and at the airport bump into a fellow classmate who is going for the same job interview. If the two are on friendly terms, they might say hi and, when they land, agree to catch the same cab from the airport to the dental clinic. If the two are on unfriendly terms, they catch separate cabs. Some job openings were widely publicised, so any student who did at least a little bit of market research could find out about them. In those cases, on the day when the employer held all the interviews, half the class would be missing at dental school. Students who did not go to the job interview would come to a lecture held on the day and exchange awkward giggles because the lecture theatre would be half empty. Some students would seethe that their friends had not informed them about the interview.

I did not like to see it. My classmates, who had got along so well for 5 years, suddenly enveloped themselves in a free-for-all hunger game, where those who were better at keeping secrets were more likely to get ahead. I thought it was ugly, and started doing something that I now believe was rather unnecessary. When I found a job advertisement that was open to new graduates, I posted it on the Melbourne Dental School Facebook page, as if making a statement to all my classmates: "There will be no secrets in this place – all information will be openly shared in collegial fashion." After graduation, I flew to Kathmandu for a 3-week volunteer trip, partly because I wanted a breath of fresh air after the gruesome final examinations and partly because it was another way to make a statement to my classmates: "I will not be part of this ugly hunger game." Looking back, I think it was unnecessary to go to such lengths to make those statements. You finish university, you look for a job – it's a natural thing for university graduates to do, even if it arouses a bit of internal competition and friction.

The prospect of working abroad in Singapore interested me when I heard that Australian dental graduates are able to practice in Singapore without sitting an additional examination. Many of my seniors and colleagues who were originally from that part of the world found employment in Singapore and told me good things about the place. I decided to go and join them. I saw it as an opportunity to experience other parts of the world and broaden my horizons. I was in my 20s, which I regarded as the Age of Exploration. *The best thing to do during the Age of Exploration, I told myself, is to explore as many places as possible and experience as many things as possible.* Before I knew it, I was on an AirAsia flight to Singapore with a series of job interviews booked.

One of my university professors was on the same flight as me. I remember thinking: she must have been a dentist for a good few decades, and she was still flying on a budget airline, travelling in a seat as squeezy as mine. It was my first moment of disillusionment as I came to the realisation that dentistry, contrary to popular perception, does not make one super affluent. Maybe I was reading too much into it. Perhaps the professor had to make last-minute travel arrangements, and a budget airline ticket was all she could find. Perhaps she just did not mind squeezy seats. But seeing her that night, on that flight, made me realise that being a dentist was not a guaranteed ticket for a smooth-sailing life, and if I wanted to afford business or first-class seats, I would have to work for it.

I found my first job in Singapore fortunately without too much hassle. My first patient, a middle-aged man in business attire, needed a dental check-up and a clean. Despite my trembling hands, I managed to finish the procedure without breaking any of my patient's teeth. *Phew!* The patient even told me after the clean that his teeth felt fresh. I felt exhilarated. I cannot remember the exact amount he paid for the session, but I could not believe that someone actually paid for the services I provided. Why would anyone pay hundreds of dollars for something that did not cost me anything? I felt the urge to tell the patient that he was my first patient ever, and that I wanted to take a photo with him, but held back the urge. Something told me that it would not have been very professional.

The first few months as a new dentist were happy times. A new graduate has no expectations, has tons to learn and is just grateful for whatever salary they earn. Just as a newborn baby is constantly amazed at everything it sees, I was constantly busy navigating my way through the new life I had found in the bustling, modern city of Singapore. I often walked by myself around Orchard Road, the main shopping district in Singapore, exploring its many shopping centres that all have distinct architectural styles and catalogues of shops. I liked to spend hours just being pushed around by the crowd and getting lost in a myriad of shops. My body was filled with a sense of invincibility that a young man feels when he has just stepped into the professional world. Full of dreams. Full of ideals. There was nothing in the world to worry about.

WHY AM I A DENTIST?

CHAPTER 3

SINGAPORE DAYS, LATTER

The first dental practice where I worked did not have a lot of patients. I saw on average 2-3 patients per day which meant that when I was at work, I was sitting idly in the back room half the time, playing with my phone or chitchatting with my colleagues. I did not mind the abundant free time at first because, as mentioned, a new graduate has no point of comparison, and after every dental procedure, I needed time to reflect on the case. But after a few months, I heard from my friends back in Australia that they were a lot busier than I was. I began to feel anxious. A full work schedule is an important ingredient for growth not just for young dentists but for any young adult entering a profession for the first time. Every day is precious during the first few years of a dentist's career, and I did not want to waste mine in an environment that offered me little impetus for growth. Of course, there is no denying that my lack of experience played a part in my appointment book being half empty. A more experienced dentist would have filled the appointment book more successfully than I did. In any case, I decided to look for a move.

The standard remuneration rates for dental associates in Singapore at the time was anywhere between 40 and 50 percent depending on the experience of the dentist. When I went for an interview at a dental clinic that became my second place of employment, they offered me 55 percent. The commission rate of 55 percent for a dental associate was unheard of in Singapore at the time, at least for new graduates barely a year out of dental school. I was thrilled that I was offered such fantastic terms, and signed the contract the day after it was offered to me. I boasted to my friends and family over Skype (Zoom was not around at the time) that I got a new job on very good terms. Alas, I was too young to realise a universal law – things that seem too good to be true always come with a hidden catch.

I found out later that my second employer ('W') had a not-so-positive reputation within the dental community in Singapore, which was why he had difficulty recruiting new dentists and had to offer remuneration above the market rate. I had not heard of W before I joined him, which was negligence on my part because I should have done some background research before I joined a new company. But as a newcomer to the country, there weren't many people around me whom I could ask for information.

At the time when I joined W's practice, he was in the middle of a financial dispute with one of his dental associates ('S'). I do not know the details of the dispute between W and S, but in any case, S wanted to leave. But S needed to find a legally valid reason to leave. At work, S scrutinised W's every move, waiting for him to take one step wrong so he could report it to the authorities and use it as a legally valid reason to void the financial obligations he had with W. When W hired me, S found an opportunity to strike.

Some legal context is necessary. Australian dentists are able to practice in Singapore without sitting an examination, but they are required to undergo a 2-year probationary period, called Conditional Registration, where the foreign dentist is required to work under the supervision of a local dentist. It is a sensible regulation in principle, intended to give foreign dentists time to familiarise themselves with the local dental scene, and attune their style of dentistry to the needs and wants of the local market.

The regulation stipulated that a foreign dentist and their supervisor must work at the same venue at all times. This part of the regulation aroused practical conundrums. What if the supervising dentist needed to go to the bathroom and leave the premises for 10 minutes? Must the foreign dentist drop all tools for 10 minutes and wait for the supervisor to return? What if the supervising dentist had to call in sick one morning? Must the foreign dentist cancel all appointments for the day, waiting for the supervisor to return to work? What if the supervisor and the supervisee are technically present at the same venue but separated by a considerable distance (for example, in a hospital building where the two individuals could be multiple floors apart)?

All ill-considered regulations undergo the same fate. Everyone interprets them differently and complies in varying degrees. Since strict compliance usually means loss of income for the business, businessowners slowly gravitate towards interpreting the rule in increasingly liberal terms.

The regulator does not enforce the rule with too much vigour as long as the intended aim of the regulation is largely being met across the board. Before you know it, everyone is following the rule de jure but ignoring it de facto. This is what was happening in Singapore at the time regarding the rule that supervisors and supervisees had to work at the same venue at all times. No one showed perfect compliance. No one.

W was appointed as my supervisor, so I had to work at the same venue as him. I admit that there were times when W and I were working at separate venues due to the practical difficulties of the regulation already mentioned. S spotted the breach and gathered evidence of the breach for months, taking photographs of staff rosters and patient records. S maintained a pleasant façade when he saw me at work, making half-hearted small talk with me and with the other staff while discreetly gathering evidence that he could use to blow up the practice. S did not have anything against me personally. His aim was to be released from the contractual obligations he had with W, even if it meant a foreign dentist had to be sacrificed as collateral damage.

When S first made reports to the Singapore Dental Council (SDC), the SDC started sending me reminders of the regulation. I showed W those letters, but he reassured me that there was nothing to worry about. "The SDC has many rules," he said, "that exist on paper but no one follows in reality." I accepted W's reassurance for three reasons. First, I noticed that many of my Australian colleagues who were also working in Singapore at the time were indeed often working away from their supervisors, reinforcing the impression that the rule existed only on paper. Second, as a newcomer to the country, I thought it best to follow the advice of a local. Different countries have different sets of unwritten industrial norms and customs, and foreign workers often have to rely on the guidance of their local employers. Third, I had joined W's practice recently and was hesitant to move jobs again, lest I garner a reputation as a 'frequent mover'. It is a stigma that is often attached to new graduates who change jobs frequently soon after graduation. An unfair stigma, I think, considering that a lot of employers are guilty of being unsupportive, or even abusive, towards new graduates during their most helpless years, forcing them to make a move.

The SDC was fed up with years of patient complaints and reports made against W, and was keen to take firm action against him while S was feeding them with concrete evidence of regulatory breaches. Once the SDC decided that the case was strong enough, they sent a letter to me and W ordering us to cease practice until the matter could be investigated. At this point, I contemplated moving back to Australia but soon realised that I was stuck in a limbo. I had let my Australian dental licence lapse when I moved to Singapore because I did not want to pay the annual licensing fee in Australia while I was away. It was a bad move. In order to renew my Australian dental licence, I had to acquire a letter of good standing from the SDC, but the SDC refused to grant me a letter of good standing while there was an ongoing investigation. When I received an email from the SDC saying that a letter of good standing could not be granted, I felt trapped. I was unsure whether I could resume work as a dentist, either in Singapore or in Australia. I felt that my entire dental career was at a crossroads.

The stress of being subject to investigation by the SDC made me do something stupid. One night, I walked into a convenience store outside my apartment. I asked for a pack of cigarettes. I am not a smoker, and had never purchased cigarettes before. I did not know any brand names. I just asked for a random brand that was printed on the wall. I think it was called Marlboro Red. I brought them home and lit one up. A few puffs into my first cigarette I felt a sudden dizziness, as if the ground suddenly shrunk beneath my feet. I put out the cigarette and went to sleep. In the middle of the night, a fit of coughing woke me up. After coughing out the phlegm, I lay in bed and felt sorry to my parents. All their life they worked hard because they wanted nothing but the best for me and my sister. During my high school years, my parents drove me and my sister to school and sport classes 6 days a week without a word of complaint. And there I was, defiling a healthy and fit body into which Mum and Dad had invested all their hopes and all their dreams. I felt disgusted at what I had done. I got out of bed and threw the remaining pack of cigarettes into the bin.

I sought legal advice. Dental Protection Limited, the professional indemnity service that I was subscribed to, appointed me a lawyer who had experience dealing with the SDC. The lawyer told me that only one strategy was effective against the SDC – to kowtow and submit. The authoritarian impulses of the SDC meant that the quicker the show of deference, the lighter the punishment would be. I saw no choice but to follow the advice of the lawyer. I was summoned to the office of the SDC, pleaded guilty, and promised not to break any rules again. I was handed an $8,000 fine for breaching the terms of my Conditional Registration. My dental licence in Singapore was suspended for 3 months. Once I had served my suspension, I could return to work as per normal. W, the main target of the SDC, received a much larger fine, and was suspended from practice for 15 months.

I later found out that W was simultaneously being investigated for a few other cases of professional misconduct. The investigation that involved me was one of many investigations he was subject to at the same time. To this day, I cannot fathom how W managed to get himself tangled into all that trouble. He really was the Jordan Belfort of the Singapore dental scene. In the subsequent months, the SDC successfully convicted W on additional charges, and he was barred from practising dentistry in his home country for a long time.

I have no grudge against the SDC. A regulatory body that oversees the dental profession of a country has the right to set up rules and enforce those rules. One may accuse the SDC of being overly protectionist and making it difficult for foreign dentists to enter the local market, but to be protectionist is a sovereign right of every country. I can complain about the procedural unfairnesses in the way the SDC dealt with me, of which there were many, but I won't. It matters little in the grand scheme of things.

The legal troubles in Singapore changed my outlook on life. I learnt that the cruelty of fate can turn one's world upside down in a way that is neither predictable nor preventable. In a funny way, I am glad that things turned out the way they did. I had gained more than I lost. I became mentally stronger. If something similar happened to me again, I would know what to do. As I said, 20s is the Age of Exploration, and any experience is good experience in the Age of Exploration.

My 3 months' suspension ended in December 2017. Fortunately, I found a new job at a different dental clinic where I could resume practice as soon as my suspension period ended. On my first day at the new job, I jested to my dental assistant that I might have "lost the touch" due to the 3 months of non-practice. The first patient of the day needed a clean. I performed the most diligent clean I had done up to that date. Something told me that every patient visit was a privilege that I should not take for granted. When the patient paid for the clean and left, I jested again to my assistant, "We have earned our daily bread, now we can go home." The assistant laughed it off, but I was serious. After months of navigating through a sea of troubles, I could finally work and make an honest day's living without fear of an uncertain tomorrow. And that is something to be grateful for.

WHY AM I A DENTIST?

CHAPTER 4

ON ORTHODONTIC TREATMENTS

In Singapore and in Australia, general dentists are allowed to do orthodontic treatments (for example, braces). Orthodontic treatments, traditionally regarded as a specialised area of dentistry reserved for orthodontists, is increasingly being seen as a new frontier for general dentists that opens up new business opportunities. In the last 10–20 years, private courses have popped up all over the world that offer orthodontic training for general dentists. Such courses are typically conducted on a part-time basis (for example, 3-day modules held every 2–3 months), which allows general dentists to attend the course on weekends. Up until the recent past, general dentists who performed orthodontic procedures were frowned upon in the dental community because they were considered to be stepping outside their boundaries. Things have changed. Now, seeking orthodontic training after finishing dental school is not only commonplace; it is considered a rite of passage. General dentists' interest in entering the orthodontic market intensified especially with the advent of Invisalign, a modern orthodontic technology that is lucrative business for any dentist who can execute it well.

It is a common belief that different areas of dentistry are legally segregated, and general dentists and specialists are only allowed to perform a range of procedures within their 'territory'. It is not possible to draw a clear demarcation between the different areas of dentistry, because all dental procedures are interdisciplinary in nature, and all dental specialties overlap considerably. There are some who believe that segregation should be legally enforced so certain treatments can only be performed by a select group of specialists. A common argument for this is that specialists are able to perform 'specialist treatments' to a higher standard (whatever 'specialist treatments' means), so segregation is in the patient's best interests. But by that logic, all resin restorations should be reserved exclusively for prosthodontists, since prosthodontists can perform resin restorations to a higher standard compared to general dentists. All cleans should be reserved exclusively for periodontists, since periodontists can perform cleans to a higher standard. There would be no work left for general dentists!

In Singapore, a locally trained orthodontist, Dr Kenneth Lew, runs an orthodontic course designed for general dentists. It is a 12-day program, conducted over the course of a year. I attended the course in 2015. I was introduced to the basic concepts of orthodontics and picked up the necessary skills to start treating simple cases. I learnt a lot from Dr Lew's course but felt that one course was not enough. I had started treating a few orthodontic cases but often felt stuck, sometimes not knowing which orthodontic wire to use for my patients, and sometimes not knowing why teeth did not move the way I wanted them to. So, I looked for another orthodontic course where I could obtain further training. Sometime in early 2016, I heard news that an Australian orthodontist, Dr Derek Mahony, was planning to convene an orthodontic course in Singapore. Dr Mahony was already running a very successful orthodontic course for general dentists in Australia and was looking to expand his business in Singapore. His new orthodontic course in Singapore was planned to be much longer in duration compared to Dr Lew's, lasting for a total of 36 days over a 3-year period. The full cost of the course was $22,400, which to a new graduate was an arm and a leg, but I considered it a worthy investment.

I attended Dr Mahony's course diligently for the following 3 years. The fact that I had sunk half of my savings into the course motivated me to absorb as much from the course as possible. I could not allow my arm and leg to go to waste! There were optional assignments in the course that students could complete for an extra level of accreditation. Dr Mahony had an affiliation with the City of London Dental School that allowed students to obtain a diploma from the school upon completing all the assignments prescribed by him. *Why the hell not?* I thought, and finished all the optional assignments.

When the course concluded in April 2019, a graduation dinner was held. Dr Mahony and the students attended. At the dinner, Dr Mahony presented me with the diploma. As he was handing me the plaque, he made an unscripted announcement to the class: among all his students who were awarded the diploma that year, in Australia and in Singapore, my marks were the highest. He followed up by saying – and I will use his exact words for historical accuracy – "This is future Dr Derek Mahony right here." To be called by one of Australia's most renowned orthodontists his potential equal was, needless to say, a great feeling.

That night also held another layer of emotional significance for me. My suspension by the SDC (Sep–Dec 2017) took place while Dr Mahony's orthodontic course (Aug 2016–Apr 2019) was ongoing. I was not allowed to work during the suspension period but was free to attend the orthodontic course as per normal. I was self-conscious in the lecture rooms during my suspension period. Although my classmates did not mention anything to me, I am sure they all knew about it – it is a small country after all. During the lectures, I avoided making small talk with my classmates. I did not want to start a conversation that could lead to people asking me about my recent happenings in life. Those 3 months really sapped my self-confidence as a dentist. At the graduation dinner, however, I was declared by Dr Mahony, in front of all my classmates, to be a meritorious student and dentist. Going home that night, with my arms full of plaques and awards, I felt a strong sense of personal vindication.

Dr Mahony may be disappointed to hear this, but I do not perform orthodontic treatments anymore. After giving it a go with a few cases, I realised that orthodontics is not my niche. Orthodontic treatments are straightforward when everything goes according to plan and teeth are moving the way you want them to move. But it is rare for orthodontic treatments, which can last multiple years, to go according to plan from the first day to the last day. Unexpected obstacles pop up constantly throughout the treatment. Teeth may refuse to move, or at times even start moving in unintended directions. Revisions and re-calibrations of the treatment plan are essential after every visit. There is an added layer of stress coming from the fact that you are treating teenagers during their most emotionally delicate years. If you screw up their teeth (and by extension, the way they look), it can leave a long-lasting impact on their physical and emotional wellbeing. For the few cases that I treated, I did my best, but after a while, I decided that orthodontics was not for me.

At the risk of sounding like a salesman, I would like to mention a textbook that helped me a lot when I first started doing orthodontic treatments: *Contemporary Orthodontics* by William Proffit. It is an authoritative textbook used in dental schools worldwide, including Melbourne Dental

School. Reading *Contemporary Orthodontics* gave me a structured understanding of the basic concepts of orthodontic treatments. I feel that too many private orthodontic courses are focused on being as practical as possible, because practicality is what attracts dentists to sign up for the course ("Attend our course, and you can start treating orthodontic cases the next day!"). But focusing on practicality comes at the cost of neglecting the theory. And theory is what enables a dentist to formulate bespoke treatment plans that meet the needs of individual patients. I found the solutions to a lot of questions I had regarding my own orthodontic cases by referring to Proffit's textbook. I say to all newcomers to the discipline of orthodontics: when you're stuck, refer to your textbook. Answers lie within.

WHY AM I A DENTIST?

CHAPTER 5

ON PATIENTS

I must have met thousands of patients over the course of my dental career. Most of them were pleasant encounters, some not so much. I rarely remember the encounters that are smooth-sailing and uneventful. It's the eventful encounters that leave a long-lasting memory. I will write down a few of those eventful episodes here, to offer a glimpse of what goes on in a dentist's head when things turn sour between a dentist and a patient.

Root Canal Treatment Cases

In my fourth year of dental school, students were given permission to start root canal treatments (RCTs) while on hospital rotations. Not long into my rotation, a patient was assigned to me who needed an RCT on her lower molar tooth. It was my first RCT on a real patient. If I could talk to the past Max, I would tell him not to choose a molar tooth as his first RCT case, because molars are decidedly more difficult to perform RCTs on compared to other types of teeth such as incisors and premolars.

That RCT took 6 months to complete. For context, most RCTs in private practice settings do not take longer than 3 to 4 weeks to complete. In my defence, there were periods when I was unable to see the patient due to university holidays, exam periods, and the patient being out of town. But still, 6 months is an absurdly long time to complete any kind of dental treatment, no matter the reason. The patient was a high school student. The poor girl had to skip school a few times so she could travel to the dental hospital in Carlton to see me. When the RCT had finally been completed, and I told the patient that it was all done, I almost felt like jumping up and down the dental room out of joy. The patient did not seem as excited as I was.

The patient was discharged from the hospital, and I did

not expect to see her again. A few months later, as I was walking past the dental hospital reception area, I noticed someone familiar sitting in front of the reception. It was the patient who I had done the RCT on. Her lower right jaw was visibly swollen, which was obvious even though I was standing about 20 metres away from her. I do not remember which side of the patient it was, left or right, where the RCT was done. I like to think that the RCT was done on the patient's left side, and the new swelling that had developed was unrelated to the tooth that I had treated, but something tells me that is wishful thinking. When I realised who it was, sitting in the waiting area, I gave a quick "huh" and attempted to briskly walk past the area. The patient turned her head, and our eyes met. I cannot forget the look that she gave me when she saw me, which was a mixture of half anger, half disappointment, half blame, and half contempt. I hope that a suitable dentist attended to her that day to manage her swelling.

My struggles with RCTs continued throughout my student days. Once, I saw a middle-aged lady for an RCT on her top molar tooth. I perforated the tooth. Perforation occurs when, during an RCT, the dentist drills too deep into the pulp chamber, resulting in a hole that opens into the adjacent jawbone. It is an iatrogenic complication – a jargon that doctors and dentists use when they are too pussy to say, "It's my fault." While it is possible to repair a perforated tooth using materials such as mineral trioxide aggregate, the long-term success of the RCT is invariably compromised.

When I realised that I had caused a perforation, I saw the Pacific Ocean unfold before my eyes. It was the first time I had caused a major iatrogenic complication on a patient. I had no idea what to do or what to say. Without saying a word, I slowly removed the rubber dam from the patient's mouth. The dental assistant helped me remove it, also without saying a word. I pressed the button on the dental chair to bring it to an upright position. The chair took about 5 seconds to make the transition, which felt like 5 years. What choice did I have? I explained slowly and calmly to the patient the events that had transpired. The RCT had to be abandoned, and an alternative treatment had to be found. After discussing the options, we decided that the tooth would be extracted at the next visit. I felt super bad.

A few days later, I called the patient to arrange the appointment where the said molar tooth would be extracted. Over the phone, the patient told me something I did not expect to hear. She asked me if she could be transferred to another dental student who was more experienced than I was. She did not sound angry or mean. She was calm and polite. It was a totally understandable request that she had made. I told her I would have it arranged. After exchanging a few more lines of meaningless pleasantries, I hung up the phone. I walked up to the dental reception area to arrange the internal referral. I don't know which dentist ended up seeing the patient. I hope she was transferred to someone more capable than I was.

Dental Bridge Case

While I was working in Singapore, a middle-aged man of French origins came to see me. Singapore is a host to many multinational corporations, and many of my patients were expatriates from all over the world. The patient I saw had a missing upper molar tooth and sought a replacement. After discussing the various options, we decided to use a dental implant to replace the missing molar. The date for the implant surgery was set.

On the morning of the surgery, before the patient arrived, I sat down and reviewed the patient's dental records. I had a look at the patient's OPG (orthopantomogram), a full-mouth X-ray that is required in preparation for surgeries of the mouth. I noticed something strange in the patient's upper jawbone where the implant was to be done. The bone around the area of the missing tooth showed a radiolucency which was most likely resorbed bone around the apex of the extracted tooth that had failed to heal. While it is possible to place a dental implant into an area of resorbed bone, the chance of success is significantly lowered. I had viewed the patient's OPG prior to that day – I do not know how that radiolucency escaped my earlier inspection of the OPG. I walked over to my boss's room and asked for his opinion on the matter. He advised me against proceeding with the implant surgery, as the risk of failure was something the patient should not have to bear. There was also a suitable alternative option – a dental bridge – the success rate of which did not depend on the quality of bone. By the time I finished the chat with the boss, the patient had already arrived, sitting in the waiting lounge. I had to break the news to him that the implant surgery could not go ahead. The patient was understandably annoyed by the last-minute change of plans but agreed to proceed with the bridge procedure.

In dentistry, when one thing goes wrong, everything goes wrong. It's Murphy's Law. The next few sessions with the patient were marred by further blunders, all of them my fault, that washed the patient's trust in me down the drain.

I started working on the dental bridge for the patient, and all the usual suspects turned up, including the temporary filling falling out at home, impressions that needed to be retaken due to inaccuracies, the bridge being ill-fitting and requiring a recall to the lab for adjustments, and so on. Dentists reading this will recognise the frustrating repertoire that always arises as a set. The patient's degree of annoyance grew with every visit, and so did my sense of dread before each appointment with the patient.

When the PVS (polyvinyl siloxane) impression for the bridge needed to be retaken for the third time, the patient got fed up to the brim. The receptionist called him to arrange an appointment, and the patient scolded the receptionist over the phone: "I will come in when I want to." A few days later, I was out for my lunch break when I received a text message from my receptionist. The patient had turned up to the dental clinic impromptu without an appointment. On my way back to the clinic, my lunch – spaghetti bolognaise I think it was – did a somersault in my belly. When I arrived back at the clinic, the patient was sitting in the waiting lounge with a disgruntled face. The clinic was designed in a way that a dentist entering the clinic had no choice but to walk past the waiting lounge and acknowledge the presence of any patient sitting there.

It's such an annoying design. Anyway, I greeted the patient as I tried to awkwardly walk past the sofa.

"Hey, we didn't know you were coming today!"

"Neither did I."

The patient's last comment was made with a sarcastic gesture: shoulders shrugged and lips pouted. I walked inside the dental room and put on my gown. I washed my hands in the basin. After patting my hands with a paper towel, I paused for a moment. I closed my eyes, drew my breath, and uttered a few words: "Dear God. Give me strength to face this patient and let the session finish without further trouble."

I am not religious, but a man gotta do what a man gotta do to muster whatever source of strength he can in times of desperation. After uttering my prayer, I walked to the waiting lounge and invited the patient into the dental room. The patient followed me into the room, had a new impression taken, and left the clinic without saying much.

In the end, the dental bridge was delivered to the patient. Even the last visit was not free of an unexpected blunder. The bridge had a high spot that needed to be adjusted, and the adjustment procedure caused a chip on the ceramic surface. I don't even remember how I tried to explain that to the patient. Needless to say, after the bridge was delivered, the patient did not return to the clinic ever again.

Denture Case

While I was working at a private dental clinic in Melbourne, a middle-aged man visited me to have a partial denture made. The patient already had a denture that he was not completely happy with, so he wanted to have a new one made. A side note about dentures is necessary. Most dentists, except a blessed few, regard dentures as the bane of their existence. It is extremely difficult to make a denture that feels comfortable. In fact, I argue that a comfortable denture does not exist, for the simple reason that you are making something rigid that is supposed to fit onto something soft. A stone pillow that is moulded perfectly to the shape of your head will be uncomfortable to sleep on. A stone sofa that is moulded perfectly to the shape of your body will be uncomfortable to sit on. Dentures are the same. The problem is that there is a considerable gap between what patients expect when they pay for a denture and what the dentist can deliver. People who pay for a denture expect, not unreasonably, something that feels comfortable in the mouth. It is something that few dentists, if any, can deliver. Although I have always struggled with dentures, I still offered it as part of my services, because dentures are a common item that patients ask for. A bartender who is bad at making martinis cannot take them off the menu, for the simple reason that they are such a frequently requested item. So, when the said patient visited my clinic and asked for a denture, I accepted the request. We exchanged pleasantries during the first few sessions. I asked him where he had his existing denture made, and that led to a conversation about the patient's past life in Zimbabwe, how he brought his five kids over to Australia, how he and his wife worked day and night to put food on the table, blah blah. It was all cordial and pleasant.

Fast forward 2 months – things had gone south. A denture was ordered from a dental lab, but it did not fit well in the patient's mouth, despite my repeated attempts at adjusting the denture. After a few frustrating visits, the patient started comparing my denture to the one he already owned. I understand when patients make comparisons. It is only natural for people to compare the present against the past, dental experiences not being an exception. Where the comparison is not applicable due to differing circumstances between the past and present, it is the dentist's job to explain that to the patient. Anyway, during a session, the patient tried to point out how the new denture was different from the old one. I tried to explain that it is natural for two dentures, made by two different people at two different times, to look and feel different. The following is an excerpt from the conversation:

"Doctor, the old denture is... (omitted). I don't know why the new denture is not... (omitted)."

"Sir, your old denture was made a few years ago, at a different lab. Sorry, I know you told me this before, but where did you say your old denture was made?"

"What?"

"Your old denture. Where did you say it was made? Where did you say you were from?"

"I'm from Australia."

"..."

Neither of us said anything. My dental assistant, who was sitting beside me, did not move a muscle. Even the computer in the room, which usually plays music in the background, had gone silent. A faint sound of the dental drill could be heard, coming from the room next door. I will not recount how the rest of the session went. The clinic ended up writing a cheque to refund what the patient had paid for the denture. From that day, I stopped offering dentures as part of my services. Patients who ask me for a denture are now sent away. I prefer to be a bartender who does not make martinis than a bartender who makes bad martinis.

I have recounted a few encounters with patients that are deep-seated in my memories. Fortunately, these stressful episodes are happening less frequently as years go by. This could be because I have learnt how to cope with stress from work, or it could be because I have become more skilful as a dentist, which leads to fewer complications and mistakes. In any case, I am glad that stressful encounters with patients do not happen so often anymore. Stress is not fun.

On Kids

Patients under the age of 5 can be a struggle. When a child of this age group does not want to open their mouth in the dental chair and starts crying, I can tell straightaway whether I (in cooperation with the parents) can successfully appease the child or not. Sometimes the child will, after a bit of wooing and begging, stop crying and start being receptive to dental treatments. Sometimes the child will be more adamant, and no amount of appeasement will be effective. It is hard to explain how I can predict the response of the child, other than to say that after experiencing enough battles, one develops a sense of distinguishing a hopeful cause from a hopeless cause.

Even if I can tell that there is no chance of appeasing a crying child, I usually put on a show of making an effort to woo the child for about 10 minutes before politely asking the parent to bring back the child another day. This is because if I declare too soon that the dental treatment cannot be done, the parent will think that I gave up too easily without even trying. "I drove my kid all the way there, and the dentist gave up as soon as the kid started crying" is what the parent will say to complain on the local neighbourhood Facebook page. So, when there is a crying child in the chair, I let the parent watch me woo and beg for about 10 minutes before I tell them with a sorrowful face that the dental treatment cannot proceed for the day.

Sometimes, a scared kid is helped out by an elder sibling during a dental visit, which creates some of the most heartwarming scenes in the dental clinic. Once, I saw a little girl, 4 years old at the time, whose dental visit was supported by two elder sisters. The three sisters, all of them no taller than the dental chair, held their hands together in a triangle while the youngest one was getting a filling done. My heart melted. Once, I saw a little boy for a clean. There was an older sister waiting in the corner of the room. When I finished seeing the boy, he ran to the older sister and hugged her. The sister started crying because she was relieved to see that her brother was safe and sound. During these moments, I feel that I am in the presence of a force that is sacred and pure.

From the age of 5 onwards, children become a lot more receptive to dental treatments. In fact, I have fun seeing kids of this age group because they can communicate effectively with grown-ups, which allows me to tease them and exchange jokes with them. Most of the time, I ask them about sport or the various happenings at school. Sometimes I push the boundary of the joke a little bit, for example, "Do you have a girlfriend?" or, "Why do you have so many freckles?" which makes the kid giggle in the dental chair. My dental assistant usually gives me a stern look when I make these jokes – I don't know why she has to be so serious.

One of the most rewarding moments practising as a dentist is seeing young patients grow into adulthood over the years. Because I recall my patients on a biannual basis, I notice when a young patient grows significantly in height within a 6-month period. When a young patient who has entered a growth spurt visits me, I often comment that they look taller, which puts a smile on the face of the accompanying parent. I like to ask these early teenage patients about their recent changes in life, for example, "Have you started shaving?" or, "Do your knees hurt at night?" For some reason, teenage patients do not look too amused when I ask these questions, and usually return a curt, one-word reply. My dental assistant then gives me a stern look, and I proceed with the dental treatment without further comments.

On Elderly Patients

In dental school, I once saw an elderly man who presented for a tooth extraction. He was either in his 70s or 80s. There was a bit of time for a chitchat while we waited for the local anaesthetic to take effect. I asked him: "Do you have any life advice for a young chap like me?"

He replied: "Do what you want to do, so you do not have any regrets." I have kept that man's advice in my heart ever since. I learnt that day that whenever I meet an elderly patient, I am making contact with a lifetime of experience and wisdom. That is why I do not hesitate to ask my elderly patients about their histories. I am always rewarded with the most fascinating stories.

The oldest patient I ever met was a Chinese lady who I treated while working in Singapore. She was either 98 or 99 at the time. She was wheelchair-bound due to her bind feet – an old Chinese custom from the Qing dynasty era. She must have been one of the last women in China to be subjected to the custom of bind feet. Her grandson, a senior himself, pushed the wheelchair for his grandmother. I was in awe. At the end of the session, I asked the grandson if I could shake the patient's hand. The grandson leant in close to the patient's ear and translated my request into Chinese. The patient, who was half deaf and half blind, nodded, and gently rested her frail hand on mine. After the patient left, I thought about the amount of endurance and resilience one would need to live through a hundred years of life. The patient is most likely not alive today. If she is, God bless her, and if she is not, may she be resting in peace.

One of the rotation programs during dental school required students to visit an aged care facility where students could provide dental treatments to elderly patients who were bedridden. It is not possible to provide an adequate level of dental service to these patients. Because the treatments are done while the patients are sitting up in their beds, the dentist's vision is impaired; because patients often have trouble breathing, any instrument that sprays water must be used sparingly; because patients cannot withstand a prolonged session, advanced dental treatments such as root canal treatments or dental crowns are out of the question. Only the basic and uncomplicated dental treatments can be done, such as cleans using hand instruments, fillings using temporary materials, and extractions.

Visiting an aged care facility for the first time was a shock for the 24-year-old Max, who had never witnessed the terminal stages of human life up close. I saw some elderly patients drowsing on the bench in the backyard. I asked one of the nurses why the patients were sleeping in broad daylight. She told me that is what they usually do – they nap throughout most of the day, only waking up for brief periods around mealtimes. She also told me that the daytime naps become longer and longer as patients get older. I wondered what the point of living would be if most of the day was spent drowsing and sleeping. I also wondered what would happen if the daytime naps became so elongated that one would sleep continuously throughout the day and night without waking. I wondered if there really existed a clear demarcation between life and death.

One of the conundrums that I often face when treating elderly patients is the issue of consent. Once, an elderly Chinese gentleman visited my dental clinic by himself. He needed a tooth extracted. The extraction was completed uneventfully, and the patient left in good spirits. A few hours later, the patient returned with two of his daughters, who accused me of performing the extraction without their consent. They complained that their father now needed a denture that they were unprepared to pay for. The father, who had been dragged back to the clinic by his daughters, looked anxious, not knowing whether to side with me or with his daughters. I replied to the daughters that it is the patient alone who has the right to consent to his dental treatments, but they did not seem to agree.

On the day when I had to argue with the two Chinese daughters, I was extra perturbed because the whole scene reminded me of my own grandmother, and a fight between her children that was related to her dental treatments. My grandmother, who is now in heaven, was in weak health during her final years of life. Soon before she passed away, she visited a dentist who told her that she needed a range of dental treatments, including a denture. A series of arguments soon broke out between the children, including my mother: "Who is going to pay for the treatments?" / "Why should I chip in the same amount when I pay for so many other things?" / "That dentist charges too much, so she should try visiting another dentist" / "It's easy for you to say when you're not the one taking time off work to take her to the dentist" / "Why does she need expensive treatments when she doesn't have long to live?" / "How dare you suggest that she doesn't have long to live" / "It's your fault that her dental health has been neglected..." I should stop, because my mother, who will read this book, will break into tears when she reads all this.

After witnessing my own mother distance herself from her siblings due to issues related to the health of my grandmother, I started being cautious whenever I propose a costly treatment plan to an elderly patient who appears to be relying on family members for financial support. I like to remind myself that a treatment plan that I casually mention to a patient can potentially lead to family feuds and break-ups. In case you haven't noticed, there are lots of things to consider when you're a dentist.

WHY AM I A DENTIST?

CHAPTER 6

ON DENTAL PROCEDURES

There are probably more than a hundred different dental procedures that I can perform. I have written down my thoughts and opinions on a select few procedures in this chapter. At the end of the chapter, I have prepared a rapid-fire commentary on a full range of dental procedures that I have experience performing.

On Cleans Without Check-Ups

Dental check-ups and cleans are two separate procedures. They have two separate item codes. The two procedures are usually performed as a set, but there are plenty of scenarios where one needs to be performed without the other. For example, some patients visit the dental clinic just to have a painful tooth checked, without necessarily looking to have their teeth cleaned. In such cases, a check-up will be done without a clean. Some patients have difficulty with plaque control, and I prescribe them a clean every 3 months (instead of the usual 6 months) which means that during the patient's every other visit, a clean will be done without a check-up.

A conundrum occurs, however, when a new patient wants to be cheeky and asks for a clean only without a check-up. Imagine that I started doing the clean procedure for a patient and noticed something in the patient's oral cavity that might interest them. In such cases, I believe that the duty to report the finding to the patient has been overridden by the patient's wish to not have their teeth examined. Exceptions could be made for clinical findings that are of vital importance to the patient, such as leukoplakia of the oral mucosa. But any clinical finding in the oral cavity can potentially be of vital importance. A seemingly small and innocuous enamel discolouration may be brooding advanced caries underneath that can potentially turn into a spreading neck infection in a short period of time. Just recently, I saw a patient who had a minor hairline crack on a lower molar, which I did not think too much of, and the patient returned a few days later with severe pain because the crack had turned out to be a lot deeper than it appeared and started turning into an infection of the lower jaw. Does this mean, then, that I have a duty to report on every hairline crack that I find, when the patient has said no to a dental check-up? Does a dentist's duty to report a piece of information override the patient's declaration that they are not interested in knowing? I do not have answers to these questions. I will leave it up to the legal experts to ponder it.

In practice, when a patient asks me for a clean without a check-up, I usually just accede to the request. If I do find things in the patient's mouth that I believe might interest them, I just tell them. I consider it added value service to the cleaning procedure that the patient has paid for. So far, I have not had a patient who said no to the added value service.

On Needles

All my patients tell me that the needle is the scariest part of visiting a dentist. The second scariest part is the bill that is presented at the end. Patients also tell me that the anticipation of pain is worse than the actual pain of getting a dental needle. The actual pain from the needle, most patients confess, is not that bad.

There are two main factors that determine the amount of pain received from a dental injection. The first factor is the rate at which the injection is given. The faster the injection, the more painful it is, and the slower the injection, the less painful. I once had to give myself an injection to numb up an ulcer in the mouth, and I made sure that the injection that I gave myself was the slowest injection in the history of injections. I am not as considerate when I inject anyone other than myself, my patients will be sad to hear. The second factor is the type of tissue where the injection is given. The tighter the tissue, the more painful, and the looser the tissue, the less painful. This is why injections given on the hard palate – where the oral mucosa is attached tightly to the underlying bone – are always more painful than, say, injections given under the tongue, where the oral mucosa is comparatively loose.

Sometimes a tooth may refuse to numb despite repeated

injections of local anaesthetic. Many explanations have been offered for why a tooth may refuse to numb, the most famous one being that a tooth with an active infection will not numb due to the acidic environment which hinders the activation of anaesthetic molecules. This explanation, while scientifically valid, is given a little too much love by dentists around the world because it is a convenient explanation that allows the dentist to blame the patient for a failed anaesthesia. I believe that, in most instances, failed anaesthesia is due not to the presence of an infection but to an inaccurately performed inferior alveolar block.

For me at least, it is the lower molars that most often refuse to numb. Lower molars require an inferior alveolar block for anaesthesia – a technique that can be tricky even for seasoned dentists, due mainly to the fact that the target nerve (inferior alveolar nerve) is located deep inside the oral mucosa. In order to hit an invisible target, the dentist has to rely on their knowledge of oral anatomy. The trouble is that the exact location of the inferior alveolar nerve varies for everyone, which means that sometimes the dentist will give the injection where they believe the target nerve to be, and miss the actual location of the nerve. When this happens, teeth that are supplied by the inferior alveolar nerve will not numb, and the dentist has no other choice but to repeat the injection until the needle finds the target nerve and the anaesthetic is deposited at an accurate spot.

I have had one patient faint in the dental chair during my 10 years of practice, and that fainting was due to the fear of the dental needle. It happened when I was working in Singapore. The patient, a middle-aged man, told me at the start of the session that he had a history of fainting at the dentist. I should have heeded his warning more closely, but thought rather carelessly that nothing would happen if I gave the injection slowly enough. After I gave the injection, the patient seemed okay, although I could see small beads of sweat starting to break from his forehead. I looked away to dispose of my dental needle. My assistant called my name. I turned to look at the patient. The patient had fallen unconscious and had started to shake violently in the dental chair.

Three different thoughts filled my brain. 1) *What is the first aid protocol for a fainting patient?* Dentists working in Singapore, including myself, receive first aid training every few years to brush up on their first aid protocols, but when an emergency episode actually unfolds in front of your eyes, all memories escape your brain. 2) *Should I call my boss, who is working in the dental room next door?* 3) But *what if he blames me for causing a patient to faint? Should I just wait it out and see what happens?*

The shaking continued for about 5 seconds. When the shaking stopped, the patient lay flaccid on the chair with arms and legs hanging loose. The patient was of Indian origins and had dark skin, but his face had become so pale that he almost looked albino. He then started snoring. My assistant and I stared at him, not knowing what to do. After about 3 seconds of snoring, the patient regained consciousness. He told me, "It's okay, this always happens when I have an injection at the dentist." Now that I think about it, it is funny that the patient tried to offer me words of reassurance, not the other way around. I needed those words of reassurance, though, because I almost felt like having a heart attack myself. I did learn an important lesson that day: the fear of the dental needle is not to be underestimated.

On Dental Crowns

Dental crowns are good money for the dentist. At the time of writing, I charge $1850 for a dental crown. It takes me roughly 2-3 hours, over two separate visits, to complete the crown procedure. Sometimes additional chairside time or additional visits are required. The lab from where I order my dental crowns typically bills me $200–300 for their works. Even if I consider the fee that is paid to the lab, and the extra chairside time that is sometimes required, dental crowns usually bring in greater revenue per hour to the dental clinic compared to most other procedures such as cleans or fillings. I call cleans and fillings the 'bread and butter' of the dental practice. Revenue generated from the 'bread and butter' procedures is usually enough to cover the overheads of running a dental practice, but it is when dentists start selling the more expensive treatments, such as dental crowns, that practices start seeing some real profit.

I feel bad using the word 'selling', but hey, this is capitalism, and private dentists are there to sell their services to their patients. The fact that private dentists must be both a clinician and a salesperson at the same time is a major source of stress for young dentists, who 1) graduate dental school with idealistic beliefs that dentists must not upsell their treatments, and 2) lack the communication skills or the chairside confidence they need to make sales pitches to their patients. When I was a new-graduate dentist, I was often called into my employer's room for a meeting because I was not generating the kind of numbers they were looking for. In these meetings when employers reproach their dentists about their financial performance, sentences such as, "You need to make more money" or, "You need to sell more treatments" are not used. Such language is too candid. Various euphemisms are used instead, such as, "You need to indicate more treatments" or, "Your diagnoses need to be more thorough." These euphemisms allow employers to say to their workhorses what the meeting is all about without saying directly what the meeting is all about.

There are online and offline courses designed to teach dentists how to sell more treatments – sorry, how to communicate effectively with their patients. I have attended a few of these courses myself at the urging of my employers who wanted to see my numbers go up. These courses certainly have their value, as effective communication is a skill that is valuable to anyone in any context. Lecturers at these courses – at least the ones who I've listened to – teach proper chairside manners and communication skills to their attendees without necessarily highlighting the link between effective communication and greater sales of dental treatments. But both the lecturers and the attendees at these courses know: the only reason the attendees are there is because they are trying to learn how to boost their numbers.

During the first few years of my career, I was bad at persuading my patients to accept my treatment proposals. The rate of acceptance gradually went up as the years went by. A number of factors contributed to my improvement as a salesman. First, I look older now compared to how I looked as a new graduate. For both male and female dentists, an appropriately aged look greatly enhances their trustworthiness in the eyes of patients, which persuades them to accept the treatment proposals made by the dentist. No one wants to spend thousands of dollars on a dentist who looks like they are fresh out of dental school. Second, my persuasion skills improved gradually over time due simply to the amount of life experience I accumulated over the years. Persuasion requires, above all, the ability to empathise with the minds of others, which only sufficient years in life can give. Third, I made efforts to study the science that justifies the use of the more expensive dental treatments, such as dental crowns. As a new-graduate dentist who lacked the necessary theory, I used to have lingering doubts in my head whenever I tried to sell dental crowns to my patients, such as: *Am I exaggerating the need for a dental crown? Am I prioritising my own financial interests above the interests of my patients?* Patients are quick to detect such signs of doubt shown by the dentist, which prevents any sales from being made. After gaining a bit of theory regarding the use of dental treatments such as crowns, I could start speaking honestly and confidently to my patients regarding their treatment plans.

Speaking of the science regarding the use of dental crowns, I do want to address one of the myths that is widespread among the dental community. Not every root canal treatment (RCT) needs to be followed by a dental crown. While the presence of a permanent restoration is important in ensuring the long-term success of an RCT, individual considerations must be given to every case, depending on factors such as: location of the tooth, the presence or absence of proximal ridges, anticipated functional load on the tooth, amount of remaining tooth structure, and so on. Also, a dental crown is not the only type of permanent restoration that can be used after an RCT. Direct resin restorations, onlays or partial crowns are all viable options. Full jacket crowns – what dentists usually refer to when they use the term 'crown' – are only one of many types of permanent restorations that can be employed after an RCT. No dental textbook or study, as far as I know, advocates a blanket rule of 'a crown after a root canal treatment'. This formula that couples RCTs and dental crowns together is recited almost as a mantra among general dentists who try to sell the two treatments as a set to their patients.

There is a reason why dentists subscribe to the formula that encourages the upselling of dental crowns. That reason can be found in the first sentence of this subchapter.

On Cleans and Deep Cleans

A lot of dental clinics offer two separate items on their menu: a regular clean and a deep clean. Give me a break. The term 'deep clean' has no scientific basis. Nowhere in the bible (*Lindhe's Clinical Periodontology*) is the term 'deep clean' mentioned. Lindhe (hallowed be thy name) does make a distinction between non-surgical periodontal therapy and surgical periodontal therapy – two procedures that are clearly demarcated by the fact that the latter involves soft tissue incision. But how do you demarcate a regular clean from a deep clean? A common answer I get from my colleagues is that a deep clean involves subgingival curettage. But my friends, a dental clean is, by definition, removal of all plaque and all calculus from both supragingival and subgingival sites. If a patient only pays for a regular clean, are you going to deliberately limit the application of the ultrasonic instrument to regions above the gingival margin, and not allow the tip of the ultrasonic instrument to dip below the gingival margin? Nonsense.

The only reason dentists separate dental cleans into two separate tiers, regular and deep, is because some cleans take longer than others, and dentists feel the need to be compensated for the amount of time they spend when cleans take extra time. This is, of course, fair enough – it is only just that people are remunerated properly for the time and effort they spend on a job. The term deep clean, therefore, exists for marketing purposes, not scientific purposes. It is an intuitive term that instantly conveys to the patient the fact that there is a lot to be cleaned; a higher fee will therefore be incurred. Due to this marketing benefit, the term deep clean will probably never be ousted from the dental menu, regardless of the scientific basis (or lack thereof) of the term. I generally disapprove of dental jargon that has been made up purely for marketing purposes. The dental lexicon is already convoluted enough as it is.

While we are on the topic of cleans that take extra time, allow me to share some extreme cases that I have had the pleasure of seeing. Stop reading if you are in the middle of a meal. Silver medal goes to a patient who I saw while I was working in Singapore. A lady in her 30s. It was clear that she had not been to a dentist for a long time, if ever. Calculus had built up around her lower premolars and molars to a point where the teeth were no longer visible. All posterior teeth had joined up and as a collective resembled the shape of, and I regret that there is no better word to describe that shape than, the Great Wall of China. Calculus had built up and joined the patient's premolars and molars in the shape of the Great Wall of China. When I saw it in the patient's mouth, I was seriously tempted to write my signature on it using my ultrasonic instrument. I didn't do it. My assistant was watching.

The heaviest calculus build-up that I have ever seen was not even from one of my patients. It belonged to a lady that I randomly spoke to, in Scotland out of all places. I was travelling in Scotland with my family a few years ago. There is an island, called the Isle of Mull, off the western coast of Scotland. It is an hour's ferry ride away from the Scottish mainland. We took the ferry and landed at Craignure – a small coastal town on the Isle of Mull. A quiet and peaceful place. Straight out of a William Yeats poem. In front of the ferry harbour at Craignure, there was an information centre. I walked into the building and saw a lady sitting behind the desk. The block of calculus that had built up around her lower front incisors had become so engorged that it was almost trying to crawl out of her lower lip.

Imagine Bubba from Forrest Gump – you get the picture. I was faced with a dilemma. Should I tell her? Would she be offended? If I told her that I was a dentist and that I could not help noticing, would she still be offended? Is it moral to ignore someone who has an obvious periodontal disease?

I ended up not saying anything to the Scottish lady. I know I am a dentist, but to her I was just a random tourist from halfway across the world. I was at a distant corner of the world, where I knew nothing about the lives and cultures of the locals. I felt out of place and out of line telling a local lady that she needed to go to the dentist. So, I kept my mouth shut. If, however, by some minute chance this book makes its way to the shores of Scotland and finds itself in the hands of a Craignure local, could someone please remind the lady working at the information centre – very gently – that she needs a dental clean. Perhaps even a deep clean.

How to Sue the Dentist

Are you unhappy with your dentist? Are you unhappy with the outcome of a dental treatment? Here is a guide for what you can do.

If you decide that you want to be a headache for your dentist, the first step is to nag them, saying you will lodge a complaint with the dental regulatory agency of your country (for example, the Dental Board of Australia [DBA]). Send an email to the dentist that lists your grievances, and mention a dollar figure that would make you shut up and go away. Most dentists will fold at this point and pay you out because 1) to be in the bad books of a government regulatory agency is what all dentists fear the most, and 2) most dentists prefer to pay to make headaches go away rather than dealing with them.

Do note that government regulatory agencies (in Australia, at least) are often concerned more about public protection than settling financial disputes between dentists and patients. The website of the Australian Health Practitioner Regulation Agency reads:

"Ahpra and the National Boards primary focus is public protection. To keep the public safe, they can take action that might affect a practitioner's registration. They can only take action against a health practitioner's registration and cannot help resolve the issue, nor arrange for compensation or the return of patient records."[1]

For example, if you report that a dentist is not following proper hygiene protocols, the DBA can order the dentist to attend courses about hygiene and take steps to ensure the dentist follows proper hygiene protocols. If, on the other hand, you report that a dentist charged you half a million dollars for a set of veneers, but you are unhappy with the outcome, the DBA will look into the matter but will not make the dentist pay you back as long as the veneer procedure was carried out safely. Therefore, if your primary concern is money, it could be faster to sue the dentist and take them to the civil court.

A courtroom is all about evidence, and nothing else matters. Also, a civil court operates under the principle of preponderance of evidence, not proof beyond reasonable doubt. This means that if you want to win a lawsuit against a dentist, the range of evidence that you present has to impress the judge more than that presented by the dentist. In most lawsuits between a dentist and a patient, the dentist has an evidentiary advantage due to the copious amounts of records they have at their disposal, such as notes, photos and X-rays. Patients on the other hand have a disadvantage due to the lack of records. The vast majority of patients will not choose to make records after every dental visit.

In order to maximise your chances in the courtroom, focus on gathering as much evidence as possible. After every dental visit, write down on your phone events and conversations that took place in the dental room. In the eyes of a judge, notes made by a patient have the same evidentiary power as notes made by a dentist. When writing your notes, use an app that records the date of entry. Do not amend a previously written note – the judge will frown upon something that has been modified. For bonus points, take photos of your teeth after every dental visit.

It could be worth visiting other dentists for third-party opinions. Do bear in mind that many dentists have the mindset of a fraternity and may refuse to say something that can put other dentists in jeopardy. Keep visiting other dentists until you find someone who is willing to give you their honest opinion without considering the interests of the fraternity.

If the dentist you are trying to sue took X-rays of your teeth, ask for a copy. Look as smiley as possible and sound as cordial as possible when you ask, because the dentist may refuse to release the X-rays if they suspect that you are up to something. Us dentists are good at smelling a litigious vibe in the air. Remember the words of the Godfather, and do not let the dentist know what you are thinking.

You signed a consent form that indemnifies the dentist against accidents and complications? Fear not, because a consent form cannot protect the dentist beyond reasonable limits. A consent form is like the terms and conditions of any other goods and services in the market – just because it contains 2000 clauses that protect the dentist, it does not mean that all those clauses will hold up in a court of law.

Most accidents and complications that happen in the dental room do not lead to a lawsuit, because the cost of bringing a dentist to a courtroom often exceeds the expected payout from a successful lawsuit. In Australia, it often costs hundreds of dollars just to have a consultation session with a lawyer, and thousands of dollars to actually go through the lawsuit process. A patient who has spent $5,000 on dental treatments and is unhappy with the outcome will choose to swallow the loss if they find out that it costs $10,000 to sue the dentist, and the chance of winning is uncertain. So, keep up those hourly rates, dear lawyer friends – we do not want to lower the bar too much for starting a lawsuit in this country, do we?

I feel that I need to state the obvious at this point. If you are really serious about suing someone, then do not listen to my gibberish, close this book right now, and call a lawyer.

Rapid-Fire Commentary on a Full Range of Dental Procedures

Code	Treatment	Comments
011	Comprehensive oral examination	Took me 200 minutes to do this as a new-graduate. Now it takes me 2 minutes.
012	Periodic oral examination	Ditto.
013	Emergency examination	Ditto, except this one takes me 30 seconds.
022	Intraoral X-ray	If I had my own practice, I would not charge extra for X-rays. It is in my interest (and the patient's interest) that I find all the cavities to fill.
037	OPG X-ray	Ditto.
113	Recontouring and polishing of pre-existing restoration	An underrated treatment that can remove overhangs that act as a plaque trap. I should do this more often.
114	Scaling	My main source of income.
117	Internal bleaching	It's necessary sometimes.
118	External bleaching	No one needs it, everyone wants it.

ON DENTAL PROCEDURES

Code	Treatment	Comments
121	Application of fluoride gel	It's good, although doing this at every single appointment for every single patient is probably an overkill.
141	Oral hygiene instruction	The single most beneficial dental procedure in the world that no dentists do, and no patients want to pay for.
151	Mouthguard	I'm a cheap-ass, so I personally just use the one from Rebel Sport.
161	Fissure sealant	It's good.
222	Periodontal debridement	See the subchapter 'On Cleans and Deep Cleans' (p66) for my thoughts on this.
311	Extraction	My favourite dental procedure.
322/324	Surgical extraction	Muahhh!
387	Replanting an avulsed tooth	Makes the dentist look like a hero.
392	Drainage of abscess	Makes the dentist look like a hero #2.
415/416	Root canal treatment – preparation of canal	Dental assistants hate this.
417/418	Root canal treatment – obturation of canal	Dental assistants hate this even more.

WHY AM I A DENTIST?

Code	Treatment	Comments
419	Root canal treatment – pulp extirpation	Dental assistants hate this, although not as much as the previous two items.
451	Removal of root filling from a previously obturated canal	I did this once, never doing it again.
511-515	Amalgam filling	Marginalised, misunderstood, misrepresented. We need justice for amalgams.
521-536	Resin filling	Amalgams were massacred to make way for these guys.
551-555	Inlay/onlay	Good treatments in theory.
556	Veneer	No one needs it, everyone wants it #2.
572	Temporary restoration	Quick and easy.
578	Restoration of an incisal corner	What 'aesthetic dentists' charge to inflate their fees.
586/587	Stainless steel crown	I don't do it. I prefer just to extract the baby teeth.
613/615/618	Dental crown	Good money, but incurs a long-term responsibility.
643	Dental bridge	Ditto.
651	Recementing crown/veneer	Not very fun.

ON DENTAL PROCEDURES

Code	Treatment	Comments
684	Dental implant, two-stage	A major advancement in modern dentistry that is serving mankind well. Will become more and more popular in the future due to the ageing population.
688	Dental implant, one-stage	A shortcut version of the previous item.
711	Full upper denture	Eww.
712	Full lower denture	Ewww go away.
721	Partial upper denture – resin base	Oh Christ please no.
722	Partial lower denture – resin base	Oh dear Lord please no!
727	Partial upper denture – metal framework	Dear Lord, why do you place upon me these heavy burdens?
728	Partial lower denture – metal framework	Shall I keep my faith in you O Lord, when you give me such dire punishments?
741	Denture adjustment	Our father in heaven, hallowed be your name.
743	Denture reline – full denture	Your kingdom come, your will be done.
744	Denture reline – partial denture	Forgive us our sins, as we forgive those who sin against us.

Code	Treatment	Comments
811	Removable retainer (after orthodontic treatment)	This is much better than 845.
825	Clear aligner (for example, Invisalign)	Should have bought Invisalign shares 10 years ago...
831	Orthodontic braces	Fun for the first 2 months, a drag for the next 2 years.
845	Fixed retainer (after orthodontic treatment)	A self-sabotage of oral hygiene.
965	Occlusal splint	It can work well if made well.

Source: Treatment codes are according to the *Australian Schedule of Dental Services and Glossary*, 13th edition.[2] Where appropriate, treatment names have been changed to layman's terms for ease of understanding.

It goes without saying that the above commentaries are my own personal private individual subjective views on the various dental procedures. It goes without saying that my own personal private individual subjective views do not represent the views of the dental profession as a whole. It also goes without saying that my own personal private individual subjective views are not intended to replace proper medical advice.

God, I hate living in a world where things that go without saying need to be said.

CHAPTER 7

ON THE DENTAL INDUSTRY

When I first started writing this book, I promised myself that I would refrain from doing two things. The first promise was that I will refrain from ranting about my personal grievances. If I do need to talk about a personal grievance, I will try to pull back as much as possible so that I am not just presenting my side of the story. The second promise was that I will refrain from being moralistic. If I do need to talk about the ugly sides of the dental industry, I will again try to pull back as much as possible so that those ugly sides can be inspected from diverse angles. As I am about to dive into the inner workings of the dental industry, I need to remind myself once more of those two promises. Remember Max, no ranting, and no lecturing. Let's see how I go.

On Conflicts of Interest

A culture exists in the dental industry where dental practices consider patients as assets they own. This is an obvious fallacy. Patients are not serfs who have pledged their loyalty to one dental practice for life. I may provide a dental clean for a patient, and the patient may leave the clinic smiling, but as soon as the patient walks out the door, it is free competition between all dentists in the market for the patient's next clean in 6 months' time. Just because I am the dentist who saw the patient last, I cannot assume that the patient will return to me in 6 months' time. The patient may seek the services of another dentist, and there could be many reasons for that. Perhaps the patient thought that my fee was too high. Perhaps the patient thought that I was too rough when I did the clean procedure. Perhaps my clinic is too far from where the patient lives. No matter the reason, if the patient did not return to see me, an unreasonable response from me would be to blame the patient's new dentist for stealing my business. It is an unreasonable response because no one can steal what I do not own. Since I do not own my patient's future appointments, I can never lose them – I can only fail to win them.

Since a dental practice is not entitled to any business generated by a patient, it follows that it is not possible for dental clinics to steal business from their competitors. Imagine that I own a dental practice, called Good Dental, in a suburb called Sunnyvale, and my clinic is the only dental clinic in Sunnyvale. Business is good. One day, another dental clinic, called Better Dental, opens next door. From that day, the number of appointments in my book starts to dwindle. I will, of course, be salty and feel that Better Dental has taken something away from me. It would be unreasonable of me to think that way. Since I never owned any of my patients' future appointments, Better Dental never took away anything that belonged to me. They merely won something that was up for free competition. Imagine there was a patient who started a series of dental treatments with me but switched to Better Dental midway through the course and finished the rest of the treatment plan with them. I would be salty, but that saltiness would be unreasonable in nature. I can always start a course of dental treatments for a patient, but as soon as the patient finishes a session, pays for that session and walks out the door, I can only hope that they were impressed enough with my services that they will return to me to continue with their treatment plan. Patients always reserve the right to their own body, and the right to choose the dentist who will touch their body. So, when the patient chooses not to finish a course of dental treatments with me, I can either curse the dentists at Better Dental for stealing my business, or start questioning why the patient decided not to finish the course of treatments with me. Tempting to do the former, wiser to do the latter.

I understand that dental practice owners cannot help but feel territorial about their business. Some of my friends are practice owners, and they pour all their heart and all their soul into running their businesses in a market that is more competitive than ever. Since I am not a practice owner, I am in a luxurious position where I can sit in high heaven and preach that dentists should suppress their territorial instincts. Yet, I maintain that territorial attitudes shown by dentists are unreasonable in nature. Imagine that I move to a rural town that lacks eligible bachelors, believe that I am entitled to date all the women in town, and declare conflicts of interest to other men who wish to move there. If a bunch of handsome men move into the same town after me, I will be super salty and feel that my territory has been violated. Such would be an unreasonable response.

On Patient Solicitations

When a dentist leaves a private group practice, practice owners become paranoid about patient solicitations. Patients and dentists often form a close personal rapport, so it is not uncommon for patients to follow their dentist to their new clinic. Practice owners hate to see this and do their best to prevent patients from escaping their grasp. I have seen practice owners eavesdrop on conversations between dentists and patients from outside the clinic room to monitor potential solicitations. I have seen practices install surveillance cameras and voice recorders in the clinic room to monitor the departing dentist's every move and every word. I have seen practices call up patients and record those phone calls in order to gather evidence of solicitation. All ugly scenes, if you ask me.

If I try to explain here why a culture of fluid patient movement should not only be allowed, but encouraged, I doubt any practice owners reading it will be convinced. But I will have a go at it anyway, because patient solicitation is one of the main sources of interpersonal conflict between dentists worldwide, which I find sad, and staying silent on the issue in this book would mean a hugely missed opportunity. Here I go:

1. When there is an ongoing treatment plan for a patient, it is best for the same clinician to continue and finish the treatment plan. Transferring an ongoing treatment plan to another dentist midway through the course is like trying to cook a dish and transferring it to another chef midway through the cooking process. It can be done, but the quality of the dish will unavoidably suffer. Transfer of patient cases can be done – it is indeed sometimes necessary – but it will take time for the new dentist to form rapport with the patient and learn about the case. Therefore, if a dental practice has patients' best interests at heart, it should make efforts to ensure that patients with ongoing treatment plans can continue seeing the same dentist. Placing a stumbling block to impede patients from finishing their treatment plan by the same dentist goes against the patients' best interests, which is not something a dental practice should do.
2. Autonomous decisions made by patients must be respected. If patients were a herd of sheep whose

ownership was attached to a single shepherd, then yes, it would be unethical, if not criminal, for a shepherd to woo a sheep that belongs to a neighbouring shepherd to jump the fence to the other side, and I would be arguing on this page against the act of sheep solicitations. But patients are not a herd of sheep, so they must be allowed to exercise autonomy and change their shepherd as often as they like. The patient may, of course, after being informed that their dentist is moving to another clinic, decide to stay with the current dental practice.

3. If the culture of fluid patient movement between clinics becomes the norm, whether a clinic loses patients upon the departure of a dentist will depend not on how obsessive the clinic is in severing all modes of communication between the dentist and their former patients, but rather on how capable the clinic is in hiring a new dentist who can bring along a large patient base. Imagine that an associate dentist leaves a clinic, followed by a mass exodus of patients. All the clinic has to do, in that case, is hire a new dentist, who will be followed by a fresh influx of patients. If the clinic has adequate pulling powers, such as modern technology, well-trained assisting

staff, and generous benefits, then it will have no problem attracting a dentist with a large patient base. Whether a clinic gains or loses patients in the long run will, in other words, depend on its merit rather than how paranoid the boss is in preventing patient departures. An industry is the healthiest when merit determines the order of success.

4. Fluid patient movement is already happening more and more with the advent of social media. Many dentists have LinkedIn profiles and Instagram pages that allow patients to easily look up and get in touch with dentists of their choosing. Most national dental governing bodies, such as the Australian Health Practitioner Registration Agency (AHPRA), make available online the registered workplace of dentists, allowing patients to easily look up the whereabouts of any dentist in the country. Transparency in the dental market and the increased ease with which patients and dentists can establish contact with each other is a wave, and in my view, a wave of progress, that can be neither resisted nor reversed.

I know it is difficult for a dental practice to start being lenient on patient solicitations. It is difficult to be the only person to line up in front of a train, when everyone else is pushing in front of you. Yet, no one will deny that the culture of lining up in front of a train is better for everyone in the long term. I ask my fellow members of the industry only to recognise that the culture of fluid patient movement is better for everyone in the long term, due to the reasons listed.

On the Code of Dental Brotherhood

There is an unwritten code within the dental community that dentists should defend each other's actions, even if it comes at the cost of honesty to the patient. It is forbidden, apparently, to say anything to a patient that portrays the patient's previous dentist in a light that is anything less than a hallowed ray of divinity. I call it the Code of Dental Brotherhood. An example is when a patient has had a dental procedure done (for example, a root canal treatment), is dissatisfied with the outcome of the procedure (for example, the tooth is still in pain) and seeks the opinion of another dentist regarding the matter. A dentist who subscribes to the Code of Dental Brotherhood will dismiss the dissatisfaction of the patient ("It's only been two months since the treatment was done, so give it more time") and downplay the negative outcomes of the procedure ("It's common for a tooth to keep hurting even after a root canal treatment").

It is a poor code that dentists must protect each other's reputation at the cost of honesty to the patient. For any healthcare professional, the duty of truth to the patient is sacrosanct. There is no need for dentists to throw each other under the bus, but at the same time, there is no need for dentists to defend each other like members of a brotherhood or a cult. Members of a profession should be collegial to one another, sure, but that does not justify lying to the patient. In the example described earlier, if the root canal treatment has indeed been performed to inadequate standards, a dentist can communicate the findings to the patient in a matter-of-fact and non-judgemental tone. Once the facts have been delivered, whatever opinion the patient forms thereafter towards the former dentist is the prerogative of the patient.

Of course, weaving words and sentences together in a way that portrays a patient's previous dentist in a neutral light is easier said than done. It is something that requires not only mastery of the English language but also a high degree of interpersonal and cultural awareness. It is something that is especially difficult to pull off for new graduates who have not yet familiarised themselves with the conventions of the industry. I have heard many stories from my colleagues where all they did was deliver facts to a patient, only to receive a phone call from a disgruntled dentist the day after because my colleague had apparently tarnished the reputation of the patient's previous dentist. A phone call like that can leave a new graduate demoralised for days. It is sad that too many dentists, upon hearing that a fellow colleague has sung anything less than a glorious hymn of praise about a previous dental treatment, jump straight to the conclusion that the other dentist must have been trying to damage their reputation. I say that there is no need for dentists to make hasty conclusions about the motivations of their colleagues.

On Burning Bridges

"I will make sure that you can't get any more jobs in this business" is a common threat that dental practice owners make to dentists who leave their company, perhaps when the breakup is on less-than-ideal terms. It is a meaningless threat that should not cause anyone to fret. Allow me to conjure up an extreme example to explain. Imagine you are a young dentist, working for a group dental practice, whose owner is extremely well-connected in the Australian dental world. Let's imagine that, after your resignation, the boss sends out a mass WhatsApp message to every dentist they know in the country, describing you as a nasty dentist who should not be hired by anyone ever again. Dentists who receive the WhatsApp message will respond in two possible ways. The first is to blindly trust the contents of the message and form a bad opinion of you based purely on the contents of the WhatsApp message. The second possible response is to take note of the message but recognise that there are always two sides to a story and reserve making any judgements about you before they have actually met you. The first response is what childish people choose. The second response is what grown-ups choose.

Now, since there are childish people in this world, and I assure you the dental world has its fair share, there will be dentists who receive your boss's mass WhatsApp message and form a bad opinion of you without ever having met you. And you know what? That is a good thing. Childish bosses have filtered you out. Next time you send your job application to a list of practice owners, children will not reply to you. Only the bosses who are mature enough to make independent judgements of you will reply, which can only be described as a good thing. Some bridges will have been burnt, yes, but the ones that are burnt are the ones you would not have wanted to cross anyway.

I know that a lot of young dentists find it hard to walk away from toxic workplaces because they fear the boss will start spreading unfair rumours that can harm their future career prospects. To all young dentists with such worries, I assure you, there are only three steps you have to take:

1. If you feel you need to leave, leave.
2. Have confidence that your future career prospects will not be affected by Step 1.
3. One day, when you become a practice owner, treat young dentists better than you were treated.

On Google Reviews

My boss at my dental clinic obsesses over Google reviews. He checks them every day to make sure the star rating stays as close to five stars as possible. I don't get it. Since my dear boss insists that Google reviews matter, perhaps my breakdown below can convince him otherwise.

1. There will always be bad reviews.
2. Online reviews are easily manipulated. I can pay a marketing company today to upload 300 five-star reviews on Google, and tomorrow the clinic will have a near perfect star rating. Restaurants, cafés

and other establishments do this all the time. Every tech-savvy customer knows – an online rating that is overwhelmingly positive is more a sign of manipulation than a sign of genuine quality.
3. A discerning customer will take note of bad reviews but will not be swayed by them, recognising that reviews are opinions, not facts.
4. Bad reputation does not lead to bad business. In fact, I would argue the opposite: most annoyingly, it's the dentists with the worst reputation who tend to thrive the most.
5. Google is one of many avenues for customer reviews, none of which are more legitimate than the other. There is certainly the illusion that Google reviews have more authority compared to, say, Facebook reviews or local community magazines, but that's just because Google is bigger. No private company that collects and displays user posts has more legitimacy than any other. My gossipy aunt, who gossips about local doctors and dentists at a local mum's club, has just as much legitimacy as a Google review which, let's be honest, is also often written by gossipy local mums.

Having said all that, I do appreciate my boss making the effort to maintain a high Google star rating. It means he cares about the business (and by extension, my income), which I should not complain about.

On Salary Withholding

When an associate dentist leaves a group dental practice, it is almost considered an industrial norm that a little bit of salary is withheld by the company for a few weeks, if not months. For example, suppose that a dentist is paid their monthly salary on the 7th day of each month. If the dentist's last day of work is on the 1st of May, then salary from 1st of April to 1st of May will be withheld. If the dentist's last day of work is on the 15th of May, salary from 1st of May to 15th of May will be withheld. Basically, any amount that the company can hold back will be held back. Things are worse when there is a lengthy notification period. Most contracts between an associate dentist and a group practice contain a termination clause that requires a 2-3-month notice period. As soon as the dentist provides notice, they cannot be certain whether any salary will be paid during the notice period.

Practice owners, of course, have an excuse for holding back the salary of departing dentists. When a dentist leaves a clinic, there are always clean-up works that need to be done. A filling done by the dentist may fall out two weeks after the dentist has left, requiring a redo. A root canal treatment done by the dentist may flare up a month after the dentist has left. Dental treatments that fail prematurely are everyday occurrences in the dental practice, and if the dentist who has done the treatment is still working at the practice, they can attend to those cases at no additional cost to the practice. But if the dentist who has done the treatment is no longer working at the practice, a different dentist has to attend to the case, which will incur cost to the practice. Since any dental treatment can fail at any time after it has been performed, clean-up works may arise months, or even years, after a dentist has left a clinic. The salary of the departing dentist that is held back by the clinic, then, acts as a 'reserve fund' that is used to pay for the cost of the clean-up works.

Withholding of money without consent is theft. Imagine you forget to pay your annual income tax, and the tax bill is overdue by 3 months. The Australian Tax Office would have every right to demand payment from you, but if they hack into your bank account and make a transfer into their account, it is theft. If you borrow $100 from your mate and forget to pay him back, your mate has every right to demand payment from you, but if he snatches your wallet by force, takes out a $100 note and tosses the wallet back at you, it is theft. If your company is obligated to pay your salary each month but refuses to pay because your departure may potentially incur cost to the practice at some arbitrary date in the future, of some arbitrary amount, it is theft. If a practice owner feels so justified in withholding salary from a departing staff member, then they can surely answer two crucial questions: How much? And for how long? Imagine that the practice owner replies: "Well, I can't know for sure, but I will hold back an amount that I deem appropriate, for a duration that I deem appropriate, and will release those funds on a date that I deem appropriate." I want to call this the mindset of a mafia, but since mafia is a strong word, and since many of my personal friends are also practice owners, I will come to a compromise, and call it the mindset of a mafia.

Associate dentists, in order to protect themselves from theft, have to resort to one of the following options. The first is to give no notice, wait for a monthly salary to be paid, then suddenly ghost the clinic. For example, if the date of payment is on the 7th of each month, the associate dentist can come to work on the 7th as per normal, look as smiley and cordial as ever throughout the day, receive the monthly salary, then on the 8th suddenly not come to work. The practice owner will seethe, quite understandably, but the most amount of salary that can be held back is the amount corresponding to the dates from the 1st to the 7th of that month. The associate dentist has, in other words, chosen to make a strategic sacrifice. The harms will fall squarely on the patients of the ghosted dentist, whose treatment plans will suddenly be up in the air. Another option that the associate dentist can choose is to enter an arrangement with the clinic where the dentist will keep returning to the clinic, perhaps once a week or fortnight, to deal with the clean-up cases. This option, while significantly more professional than the first, is only possible if the dentist continues to reside in reasonable proximity to the clinic. The need to make return appearances restricts the dentist's future choice of residence and employment, so is not always feasible. Also, neither the dentist nor the clinic is obligated to enter the arrangement of return appearances. Contract ended is contract ended – all parties of a business contract should be able to terminate a contract according to its terms and walk away from it without having to enter a fresh arrangement.

It would be nice to see the dental community come up with a solution that is professional, respectful to all parties involved and fair to all parties involved. I would like to offer one: make it an industrial standard to insert a clawback clause in the employment contract between the associate dentist and the dental practice, specifying the amount and duration of withholding. Since it's the withholding of money without consent that associate dentists (and frankly, anyone) find offensive, spelling it out in the employment contract will eliminate the source of offence. Imagine that a contract between an associate dentist and a dental practice stipulates an amount of $10,000 to be held back for 2 months after the dentist has left. During the 2-month period, the total cost of clean-up works may stay below $10,000 or exceed $10,000. It is something that no one can predict for sure, so both parties can consent to taking on an equal amount of risk and shake hands on it. I am not saying that $10,000 is the appropriate dollar figure to be withheld. It is something that can be negotiated at the time of hiring.

That reminds me. I owe someone an apology. After finishing dental school, I went for a job interview at a dental practice in Sydney. The owner offered me a contract which included exactly what I described – a clawback clause that would hold back a sum of money if I left the clinic within 12 months of hiring. At the time, such clawback clauses were a rarity. I had gone to a few different job interviews, and none of them offered me a contract that contained such a clause. I called up a few mates who were also looking for jobs at the time. None of them had heard of a clawback clause. I declined the contract that was offered to me. The owner asked me why. I told him I did not know what to make of the clawback clause. The owner tried to explain the rationale to me, but I thought he was just trying to justify something that was outside the industrial norm. After 10 years of being in the trade, I now understand that a clawback clause is a fair and professional way of deciding what will happen when a practice-dentist relationship does not turn out to be as rosy as everyone hopes at the start. I say sorry to the practice owner in Sydney who offered me a contract that was completely fair, but was dismissed by an infant dentist who had no idea what was going on.

Talking about and negotiating exit clauses at the time of hiring is, of course, uncomfortable for both the dentist and the practice. It is like a couple talking about and negotiating the terms of divorce as they discuss their wedding plans. No dentist likes to say to the clinic, at a job interview, "When I leave, I want the notice period to be as short as possible." No practice likes to say to the dentist, at a job interview, "When you leave, we will hold back ten thousand dollars for three months." These are uncomfortable chats, but they are better had than not. I believe that as clawback clauses become more widespread, talking about them at job interviews will not feel so awkward anymore.

I have a personal policy. When I leave a clinic, and my salary is being withheld, I do not chase it. You see, my hair has recently started to recede, and according to my calculations, the cost of getting hair implants to replace the hair that I could lose due to stress is greater than the amount of salary I could retrieve by chasing after it. Whenever my salary is withheld, I casually tell myself that it is the cost of relocation, and try my best not to think about it, so my stress hormones do not reach my hair follicles. Other dentists may respond differently when their salary is withheld – it is their decision. I would, however, like to advise all young dentists reading this: whatever choice you make, please please please do not ghost your patients by suddenly not turning up to work one day. It's just not nice.

On the Future of Dentistry

The following is a rant about AI taking my job.

The replacement of human dentists by robots with artificial intelligence, I think, is inevitable. And I believe it will happen sooner than everyone expects. I say that human dentists have at most 20 years left, the last 5 of which will be marked by a gradually dwindling patient flow as patients flock towards AI dentists. This book may be the last memoir ever published by a human dentist.

I asked ChatGPT whether dentists will ever be replaced by artificial intelligence. The following is the response I got:

> **Me:** *Will dentists ever be replaced by AI?*
>
> **ChatGPT:** While AI is advancing rapidly and has the potential to revolutionize many aspects of dentistry, it is unlikely that dentists will be completely replaced by AI... (omitted)... the human element of dentistry – such as manual dexterity, patient interaction, personalized care, and decision-making in complex or unexpected situations – cannot be easily replaced by AI.[3]

ChatGPT says the human element of dentistry and personalised care cannot be replaced by AI. But there is something that ChatGPT, dare I say, is overlooking. We have an entire generation of kids growing up who are learning to distance themselves from the human touch. They do not pick up phone calls, even from people they know. At a restaurant, they prefer to order food using an iPad rather than with a waiter. Social media is their playground. All university lectures are now conducted online. Even I am not immune to this global trend of reduced interpersonal interaction. When supermarkets first introduced self-checkout kiosks, I hated them, but now I prefer them. They're just more convenient.

You think dental patients 20 years later will prefer to be seen by a human dentist because they desire the human touch? No chance. Patients in 20 years will far prefer a dental machine that can be asked 10,000 questions without being annoyed, and answer 10,000 questions without making a single mistake. A robot dentist will, in a matter of minutes, if not seconds, identify all carious lesions and periodontal pockets in the oral cavity, and print out various treatment options, all with quotations accurate to the last cent. Patients will value the sense of control over their own body and finances, even if it comes at the cost of sacrificing the human touch. During restorative procedures, cavity preparation will be done with a level of precision not achievable with the human eye, and during clean procedures, all plaque and calculus will be removed to a level of meticulousness not achievable with the human hand. Manufacturers of robot dentists will, at first, have to charge a fee that justifies the initial costs of research and development, but that will lessen over time as the market matures.

I think the only major hurdle to the spread of robot dentists is the medico-legal side of things. If a robot dentist breaks down during a dental procedure, as machines do, and injures the patient, who pays? As soon as lawmakers can figure that out, robot dentists will roam the earth, and kick human dentists like me out of business. And on the day when I am forced to shut my dental clinic because no one wants to visit human dentists anymore, I, like my father and forefathers before me, will grumble that ageless line: "Things were better back in the day."

CHAPTER 8

MONEY MATTERS

People think dentists are rich. I have never thought of myself as a rich person. Comfortable, maybe, but not rich. Dentists, like everyone else, must every day navigate through the myriad of rules, conventions, nuances, and interpersonal diplomacies of a capitalist society to stay afloat. At the risk of being accused of whinging, I will illustrate in this chapter the various conundrums that dentists face every day regarding the financial side of their careers.

How Much Do/Should Dentists Make?

This is the amount of money I made (pre-tax), working as a dentist, in the past 4 financial years:

FY2020-2021: $195,387

FY2021-2022: $146,593

FY2022-2023: $167,122

FY2023-2024: $169,356

I have a 40:60 arrangement with my company, so the above figures are roughly 40 percent of the total amount that was billed to my patients. The above figures do not include the various types of government subsidies that were given out during the COVID-19 pandemic. The drop between FY20-21 and FY21-22 is due mainly to a reduction in the number of working days, from 5 days a week to 3 days a week. The above are pre-tax figures. I have included a table of Australian personal income tax rates of FY2023-2024 for reference.

I usually qualify for either the highest income bracket ($180,001 and above) or the second-highest income bracket ($120,001-180,000), which means that my income tax rate usually lies somewhere between 30 and 40 percent of my pre-tax income.

Resident tax rates 2023-24

Taxable income	Tax on this income
0 – $18,200	Nil
$18,201 – $45,000	19c for each $1 over $18,200
$45,001 – $120,000	$5,092 plus 32.5c for each $1 over $45,000
$120,001 – $180,000	$29,467 plus 37c for each $1 over $120,000
$180,001 and over	$51,667 plus 45c for each $1 over $180,000

Source: Australian Taxation Office.[4]

My figures are, of course, not representative of dentists nationwide, whose work and life circumstances vary widely. Dentists who are less experienced than me will likely earn lower figures. Dentists who perform advanced dental procedures such as dental implants will likely earn higher figures. It is difficult to provide a single number that answers the age-old question that everyone likes to ask: "How much do dentists make?" I have disclosed my own figures just to give everyone a rough idea on the earnings of a general dentist who has been in the trade for about 10 years.

A question that is even harder to answer is this: How much money should dentists make? In other words, how much should dentistry cost? I believe that in the free market economy, there is no such thing as how much something should cost. Whatever the consumer is willing to pay for a good or a service is how much that good or service should cost. As long as there is enough fluidity in the market, the power of the invisible hand will ensure that the price of dentistry does not rise to a level that is unaffordable for patients, and not fall to a level that is unsustainable for dentists. If the cost of dental services is too high, there will be a net entry of dentists into the market, and the abundance of supply will eventually push down the average price of dental services. If the cost of dental services is too low, there will be a net exit of dentists from the market, and the scarcity of supply will eventually push up the average price of dental services, until an equilibrium is reached.

Caveats of course apply when discussing the economics of healthcare. Unlike most other goods and services, dental treatments have no external competition. If the price of Netflix is too high, I can switch to other modes of entertainment, such as PC games, or going to the movies, which forces Netflix to think twice before raising their monthly subscription fees. But if I have a toothache, and the price of dental services is too high, I have no choice but to go to the dentist. The traditional rule of economics that the availability of alternatives suppresses the price of goods and services is qualified when it comes to healthcare. Also, even a month's window when the price of dental services stays above the equilibrium is intolerable for consumers. If house prices are too high, I can potentially wait for months, or even years, until house prices come down before I make a purchase. But if I have a toothache and the price of dental services is too high, the most I can wait is probably a month, if that. The traditional rule of economics that high price drives away demand until price is lowered is also qualified when it comes to healthcare. If I have a son who has a dental abscess but the cost of visiting a dentist is too high, I am not going to tell him, "Have faith in the power of the invisible hand, my son, we just need to wait for people to recognise the fact that dentistry is currently overpriced, which will lead to more dentists entering the market, which will intensify internal competition within the dental industry, which will eventually push down the price of dental visits. That is when I will take you to the dentist." Adam Smith himself is not going to say that to his own child. For these reasons, I believe healthcare to be an industry where a deviation of price away from the equilibrium, especially an upward deviation, must quickly be restored, through artificial intervention if necessary.

Still, the invisible hand of the free market must be allowed to reign as the primary determinant of the cost of dental services, as it is the most effective way to ensure the long-term viability of the dental market. For the invisible hand to function effectively, factors that generate friction in the movement of prices in the dental market must be kept in check, such as: dental clinics impeding fluid patient movements (discussed in Chapter 7), lack of transparency in the cost of dental services, and gatekeeping actions by the existing dental community that suppress the entry of new dentists into the market. These are all things that might profit individual dentists in the short term but are detrimental to the health of the dental market in the long term.

I will try coming up with a fair figure for the price of dental services, using my personal circumstances, and I repeat, my personal circumstances, as a guide. For me, the minimum amount of post-tax income that will persuade me to stay in the dental industry is about $8,000 per month. A figure lower than that will not only be insufficient to compensate for the initial investment I made to become a dentist (that is, dental school tuition fees and the opportunity cost of 5 years of study), but will not be enough to cover the ongoing costs of practising as a dentist (that is, licensing fees, indemnity costs, costs of continuing professional development). For me, the minimum income threshold is $8,000 per month, but this figure will be higher for dentists who have various financial commitments. I do not have kids. I am a simple man who drives a Hyundai and does not wear a watch. I say, therefore, that my minimum income threshold of $8,000 per month is on the low side. In any case, taking $8,000 per month as the minimum income threshold, it is possible to go through a process of reverse engineering to establish the amount that I need to bill my patients per working hour:

- $8,000 post-tax income
- $12,000 pre-tax income (taking 33 percent as the personal income tax rate)
- $30,000 monthly billing (taking 40 percent as the commission rate)
- $1,500 daily billing (assuming 20 working days per month)
- $214.30 hourly billing (assuming 7 working hours per day)

$214.30 is the minimum amount that I need to bill my patients, per hour, for me to stay in the dental business. This is a figure that will allow me to make ends meet without making any savings. If life one day throws me a curve ball, such as it does, and I am faced with an unexpected large expense (for example, medical bills, lawsuits, or the car breaking down), I will be done for, since I will not have any savings. I therefore need to bill a bit more than $214.30 per hour to ensure my long-term survival. A more realistic figure would be $300 per hour. Since a typical dental check-up and a clean for an adult patient takes me 45 minutes to complete, they should cost $300 × 0.75 = $225. Yup, that sounds about right. This is roughly how much I actually charge my adult patients for a check-up and a clean. Hooray! I have been neither overcharging nor undercharging my patients. I told you that the power of the invisible hand always picks the right number for the price of goods and services.

On Dental Tourism

Every once in a while, I have patients who present at my clinic with all of their teeth splinted together with long-span ceramic bridges. These long-span bridges always have multiple design flaws that lead them to destined failure.

I won't bother going through those design flaws here – I would not know where to start. The story told by these patients is always the same: "I was overseas for a holiday. I visited the local dentist to get all my teeth done. I came back, and now everything hurts." I discover, upon examination, multiple long-span bridges that are failing due to the deteriorating health of the supporting teeth. There is often not much the dentist can do in such cases. The only viable option is to extract all affected teeth and replace them with dentures. When I tell these patients that the long-span bridges have to go, they usually enter a state of denial, refusing to believe that the dental work they got done just a few months ago could fail in such a short period of time.

I do not want to name the countries where these long-span bridges are usually made, because honestly, I have seen them hail from countries all over the world. The countries that produce the long-span bridges do have something in common – dentistry is sufficiently cheaper than in Australia to a point that facilitates a market for dental tourism. Suppose that it costs $5,000 for a 2-week holiday in a country of your choice, and it costs $5,000 to get 'all your teeth done' while staying in that country. Also suppose that it costs $20,000 to get the same treatment done in Australia. It would be naïve to not expect patients to consider the option of purchasing dental services overseas while on a holiday.

An unfortunate consequence of Australia being a net exporter of dental patients/tourists is that a sense of elitism – bordering on racism – has taken hold among the Australian dental community. On online forums for Australian dentists, the term 'overseas dentistry' is synonymous with 'bad dentistry'. This is obviously a gross generalisation. You cannot put the entire world minus Australia into the same basket and call it bad. There are plenty of Australian dentists who perform subquality works – just thinking about some of them makes my blood boil – and there are plenty of dentists around the world whose superb craftsmanship puts many Australian dentists to shame. Generalising statements such as "overseas dentistry is bad" are as unfounded as they are arrogant, so I would like to discourage my fellow Aussie dentists from saying such things, even in jest.

Consumers cannot be stopped from travelling overseas in search of cheaper goods and services. It is an inevitable economic phenomenon that cannot (and should not) be resisted. All I can do as a service provider is remind my patients that cheaper services come with risks. I am reminded of a poster that I saw once, hanging in a pub, that I would like to share: *Good and cheap will not be fast, good and fast will not be cheap, cheap and fast will not be good.* It is a mantra that Australian consumers – including myself – would do well to remember. Perhaps I should get a copy of that poster and hang it in my dental clinic.

On Quotas

In 1936, Joseph Stalin ordered the start of the Great Purge in the Soviet Union. Instructions were sent across Siberia that contained quotas for arrests and executions. Regional party officials had to meet those quotas, lest they be sent to the Gulags themselves. When insufficient numbers of 'real' criminals were found, party officials started arresting and executing anyone and everyone they could find to meet their quotas. Millions of innocent lives were lost.

I trust that the historical example described above is enough to demonstrate the dangers of quotas. They have no place in the healthcare industry, period. Imagine, for example, that a monthly revenue quota is imposed on dentists in a private group practice. Since there are always seasonal and monthly fluctuations in the number of patients that visit the dental clinic, it is only natural that in some months, revenue generated by a dentist will rise above average, while in some months, revenue generated by the same dentist will fall below average. But when a quota is in place, then in the months where revenue generation is falling below average, a force will be created that will pressurise the dentist to engage in overdiagnosis and overtreatment for the remainder of the month, so the prescribed quota can be met by the last day of the month. Overtreatment, I hope everyone will agree, is an ancient enemy of all healthcare professionals and all healthcare industries. Therefore, any force that makes the dentist more likely to engage in overdiagnosis and overtreatment should be stamped out as soon as it is identified.

Imagine that you have a heart condition and visit a heart surgeon to discuss the possibility of undergoing an open-heart surgery. The heart surgeon advises you that a heart surgery is a good idea, so you agree to it, and set the date for the surgery. As you are about to leave the cardiology clinic, you overhear a conversation coming from the doctor's room – "*Phew*, I can meet the quota for the number of heart surgeries I perform this month!" Needless to say, your trust in the heart surgeon, and the cardiology industry in general, will be destroyed. If heart surgeons should not have quotas on the number of hearts they cut open per month, why should dentists be allowed to have quotas? As wise people have said – what you do not want done unto you, you must not do unto others.

On Government Subsidies and Private Insurances

Dental treatments are expensive, so most countries have government subsidies that help their citizens pay their dental bills. In Australia, we have the Child Dental Benefit Scheme which subsidises the cost of dental treatments for patients under the age of 18. We used to have the Chronic Disease Dental Scheme which had to be closed in 2012 due to loopholes that were heavily exploited by dentists. In Singapore, they have government schemes such as the Community Health Assist Scheme (CHAS) and the Medisave scheme that subsidise the cost of dental treatments of Singaporean citizens. In addition to these government-funded schemes, a lot of patients also take out private dental insurances.

It is easy for dentists to make excessive or fraudulent claims to public dental subsidy programs and private dental insurance companies. One big reason for this is that diagnosing dental diseases or assessing the complexity of dental procedures is subject to the opinion of the dentist, so it is easy for dentists to exaggerate the gravity of dental diseases or the complexity of the procedures they perform in order to make claims that are attached to a bigger dollar sign. When patients pay their own fees, the dentist is at least to a degree disincentivised from engaging in overdiagnosis or overtreatment, because if the fee is too high, the patient won't pay. But when the government or the insurance company is paying, there is nothing stopping the dentist from going wild and making as many diagnoses as possible. And patients are usually happy to go along with it because everyone wants to maximise the benefits they get from the government or from their insurance company.

To demonstrate some examples, I will talk about CHAS, a public scheme in Singapore designed to help patients from lower socio-economic backgrounds, and AIA, a private insurance company in Singapore that provides dental coverage for its members. I hesitate to use these examples from Singapore because it makes Singaporean dentists look bad, but CHAS and AIA are the programs that I have had the most first-hand experiences with, which allows me to describe the way they work in close detail. It goes without saying that exaggerated and fraudulent insurance claims happen in every country, including Australia.

When I first arrived in Singapore, CHAS was in its infancy, and many of its terms and conditions were poorly defined, leading to loopholes that were taken advantage of by local dentists. For example, the scheme provided different levels of subsidy for a 'simple filling' and a 'complex filling'. The amount of subsidy was around $30 for a 'simple filling' and around $60 for a 'complex filling' (I cannot recall the exact dollar figure). Since the scheme did not provide any guidelines on the difference between a simple filling and a complex filling, every dentist in the country started arguing that their fillings were complex in nature so they could claim the higher level of subsidy.

I once had an argument with my boss because I thought the item 'complex filling' should not be claimed 100 percent of the time. If every filling is complex, then what filling is simple? After the argument, I continued to claim 'simple filling' for fillings that I personally regarded as being simple to perform. One day, I walked into the boss's office to ask him something. He was out for lunch. I noticed some paperwork lying on his desk. It was the CHAS claim forms that I had filled out earlier for the patients that I had seen. The item 'simple filling' had been crossed off by someone, and the item 'complex filling' filled out instead. The higher level of subsidy had been claimed from CHAS. The following month, I checked my payslip, which contained the list of dental procedures that I had performed the previous month. I noticed that I had been paid the amount corresponding to 'simple fillings'. My boss had claimed for 'complex fillings' from CHAS without telling me and paid me out for 'simple fillings', pocketing the differential amounts for himself. I was not very happy.

AIA is one of the popular private dental insurance companies in Singapore. The dental benefits provided by AIA for its members were generous, but the claim form they asked dentists to fill out contained linguistic ambiguities that were open to exploitation. For example, the list of dental procedures that were covered by AIA contained two separate items:

- 'Prophylaxis – Routine (Scaling & Polishing)', claim amount $43
- 'Complex Prophylaxis/Fluoride Treatment', claim amount $60

It makes you scratch your head. What if you did a routine clean for a patient and did fluoride treatment afterwards? Which item do you tick? Singaporean dentists decided that they should tick both items. What if you did a clean that you thought was complex, and did fluoride treatment afterwards? Dentists claimed the second item twice.

The form also contained the following two items:

- 'Tooth Extraction', claim amount $30
- 'Surgical Extraction – Erupted Tooth', claim amount $140

Dentists started arguing that all tooth extractions are surgical in nature (this is technically true, by the way), and always claimed the latter item, and never claimed the former. In the absence of clear guidelines on which item should be claimed in certain situations, everyone gravitated towards interpreting the form provided by AIA in a way that maximised the amount they could claim.

I was annoyed. I like things to be clear, even if that clarity comes at a personal cost. Once, my ex-girlfriend's landlord forgot to send her the water bill for many months. She told me to keep quiet, but I sent the landlord a polite email to enquire. The forgotten water bills were sent to us a few days later. My girlfriend was furious. She made me pay those bills. In a similar vein, when I saw that the AIA claim form contained linguistic ambiguities, I could not help myself and made a phone call to the AIA company to ask for some clarifications. The lady on the phone was nice and was happy to answer my queries. One clarification that I got from the phone call was that after doing a clean for a patient, only one of the two aforementioned items –

'Prophylaxis – Routine (Scaling & Polishing)' or 'Complex Prophylaxis/Fluoride Treatment' – could be claimed, but not both.

There is a Facebook group for dentists working in Singapore. The night I made the phone call to AIA, I uploaded a Facebook post on the group page, summarising what I had learnt from the call. I wrote in the post how some items on the claims list are mutually exclusive, so only one of them could be claimed at a time.

Soon after I uploaded the Facebook post, I received a phone call from an annoyed Singaporean dentist who I knew personally. He scolded me for, well, I still do not know what the scolding was about. It was something along the lines of, "You shouldn't tell people that stuff. I know it's fairer for everyone, but don't tell other people." It was clear that he was also benefiting from the loopholes of the AIA insurance and wanted the terms of the insurance policy to remain ambiguous and exploitable. I do not know why he or my ex-girlfriend had to scold me for trying to bring some clarity and honesty to this world.

CHAPTER 9

ON HAMLET AND DOENJANG-JJIGAE

In January 2020, news started circulating that a deadly virus had appeared in China. It did not take long for Coronavirus-19 to land on Australian shores. Public outrage was directed towards a general practitioner working in Toorak, who came into work despite having cold symptoms in the morning and was later diagnosed with the COVID-19 infection. Vitriol was also directed at a teenage girl who drove from New South Wales to Victoria, carrying the virus with her. I thought it was unfair to throw stones at these individuals, given that the spread of the virus was an inevitability.

As the COVID-19 infection started spreading out of control, the government started shutting down businesses, sector by sector. The dental community waited nervously for a government directive. Some dentists argued that dental clinics should be shut in order to join the nation-wide effort to curb the spread of the virus. Some dentists argued that dental clinics provide essential services to the public, so should remain open. The former accused the latter of being irresponsible. The latter accused the former of being irresponsible. There is a Facebook group called Dental Product Review (DPR) where Australian dentists upload posts and exchange opinions. Needless to say, DPR was on fire during the early weeks of the pandemic.

The dental profession in Australia is overseen by the Australian Health Practitioner Regulatory Agency (AHPRA) and the Dental Board of Australia (DBA). Both organisations were slow in deciding how dentists should respond to the pandemic. It was the Australian Dental Association (ADA) that first published a list of recommendations to Australian dentists. The ADA recommended that dental practices could stay open during the pandemic but should only provide emergency procedures such as extraction of an abscessed tooth, and defer any non-emergency procedures such as cleans and teeth whitening. But the ADA is no more than a gathering of dentists, and any announcement made by it lacked legal authority. Whatever the ADA recommended remained just that – a recommendation. Therefore, the arguments on DPR raged on. Some dentists argued that the ADA had made a sound set of recommendations that should be followed, especially in the absence of a legally binding directive from the government. Some dentists argued that the ADA is no more than a group of senior dentists in the country, and it should be up to individual practices to decide whether to listen to their recommendations. Arguments of both sides had merit.

Eventually, on 25 March 2020, the Department of Health made an announcement that it would adopt the recommendations of the ADA as a legally binding national policy. That settled it. Dental clinics nationwide would, for the time being, only provide emergency procedures. The clinic I worked at also followed suit. The majority of patient appointments were cancelled or deferred. Since business was expected to be a fraction of what was normal, a temporary work schedule was created that distributed the limited number of work shifts among dentists and dental assistants. A lot of dental assistants struggle to make ends meet, so the number of working hours per week is a sensitive issue for them. While everyone understood that there had to be a massive cutback on the number of hours, employers had to make sure that the hours that were available were evenly distributed among the staff. My days were also cut back, so I only had to come into work 1-2 days per week.

On 31 March 2020, the Victorian government announced the start of Stage 3 Restrictions – otherwise known as the 'lockdown'. During the lockdown period, people were only allowed to leave their homes for essential purposes, such as buying groceries or going to the hospital. It was the first of many lockdowns to come.

Like many other Australians who were out of work, I was at first optimistic, almost jovial, about the lockdowns. I saw the lockdown period as an unexpected holiday, when I could catch up on house chores and gardening. It was a chance to do some reading at home. I had always been an introverted person, so I did not think that lockdowns would be a problem for me. I was wrong. About 5 days into the first lockdown period, gloom and lethargy set in.

I opened my eyes in the morning and realised that there was no reason to get out of bed. I stared at the ceiling, rolled in bed, fidgeted with my phone, checked on Facebook how the global economy was falling apart, got out of bed, got some food in my belly, crawled back into bed and continued fidgeting with my phone. After a few days, I realised, to my dismay, that this is how life will be when I retire from dentistry in the future.

During the lockdown periods, the Victorian government gave out subsidies to people who were out of work. I qualified as a recipient. The subsidy payments were nowhere near the level of my regular income from dental work, but enough to pay for my food and everyday expenses during the lockdown period. The fact that my basic necessities were covered by the government was good and bad. Good because, well, it was free money, and bad because it forced me to ask myself a scary but important question – what would I do with my life if money and basic survival were not an issue? The only answer I could give was, "Not much." But if there is not much to do with your life, what is the point?

I did not realise at the time, but looking back, I was showing signs of mild depression. I started questioning the meaning of work and life. *Why work? What is the point? Why live?* It did not help that the first book I decided to read during the lockdown period was Shakespeare's *Hamlet*, because in the play, Prince Hamlet throws the exact same question to the audience – "To be or not to be, that is the question." It also did not help that I am naturally fascinated by topics such as the meaning of life, so when I started having morbid thoughts, I did not tell myself to stop, but encouraged myself to look directly into the abyss. It was a rare opportunity to have an honest conversation with myself about the big questions in life. These questions went away eventually when the lockdown periods ended and work resumed as per normal. If work does not provide answers to the big questions in life, it can certainly act as a good distraction and prevent one from asking those questions.

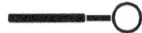

The Victorian government shut down the majority of businesses in the state. An air of apprehension engulfed the city. One needed a valid reason to leave the house. One day, I had to go into the CBD to buy something. It wasn't an essential item, but I told myself it was. On my way to the city, in the train, I rehearsed a story that I could tell the police in case I was stopped and questioned. When I stepped off the train at Melbourne Central Station, I discovered a city that was bleak and depopulated. For some reason, the sky seemed scarlet red, reminiscent of William Strutt's painting of the 1851 Black Thursday bushfires. Stores were covered with steel folding gates. Lights were on, but no customers or staff, except maybe a lone store manager inside JB Hi-Fi or Foot Locker who came in to organise the inventory behind closed doors. There were a few police officers patrolling the corners of streets. Pedestrians avoided making eye contact with the officers and walked around them to prevent being questioned about why they had to be in the city. It was a scene straight out of a dystopian film.

Yet among the general sense of doom and gloom, I noticed hints of optimism and hope. An advertisement board in Melbourne Central displayed *Hang in there Melbourne!*, like a banner held up by a soldier on a clouded battlefield. The vibrance of the city that Melbournians are so fiercely proud of had gone dormant, but not extinguished. The city was eagerly and patiently waiting for the day of liberation when it would spring back to life.

I accidentally bumped into two police officers as I turned a corner. I was petrified at first, as the story I had rehearsed on the train evaporated in my head. But instead of asking me interrogative questions, the officers gave me a thumbs up and allowed me to walk past them. It was as if the police force as a collective understood the general hardships suffered by the citizens, and determined not to stress them any further. Instead of being interrogative, the police officers seemed to give the people on the streets the benefit of the doubt. I am grateful for the empathetic attitude and the level of professionalism shown by the Australian police force during the COVID-19 pandemic. It would not have been an easy job for them, either.

As an additional measure to contain the spread of the virus, the Victorian government implemented a 'Ring of Steel' around the city of Melbourne. The policy was aimed at quarantining the entire city in a bid to prevent cases from spreading to rural Victorian regions that were still relatively unaffected by the pandemic. Freedom is a funny thing. Before the pandemic, when I was free to drive anywhere, I would very rarely travel outside my immediate vicinity, but knowing that the city was under a travel ban suddenly aroused a strong desire to escape and test the boundaries of my freedom.

I believe it was in the middle of the second or the third

lockdown. It was a day when I was not rostered to work. I got into the car and started driving.

This was my plan: I wanted to do a drive from Melbourne to Ballarat. There was no special reason why I chose Ballarat as the destination of my escapade. It was a medium-sized rural city, about two hours' drive from home (western Melbourne), that just felt like a suitable destination. Since Melbourne was surrounded by a Ring of Steel, and every road exiting the city had a police checkpoint set up, I needed to come up with a legitimate-sounding excuse to pass through the checkpoint. Luckily, I was working part-time at a dental practice in Geelong at the time. People who lived in Melbourne but had work outside the metropolitan boundary were exempt from the Ring of Steel. I was not rostered to work in Geelong that day, but the police did not have to know that. I packed some documents in my bag that could prove my employment in Geelong. To give credence to my excuse, I had to drive through a checkpoint in the direction of Geelong rather than Ballarat. Instead of driving in a straight line in a northwest direction from Melbourne to Ballarat, I had to head southwest towards Geelong first, pass the checkpoint, then turn my car towards Ballarat. It would be a detour of around an hour, which I did not mind. My main concern was how rigorous the police would be, at the checkpoint, in questioning the details of my excuse. Would they require proof that I was actually rostered to work in Geelong on that day? I did not think they would, but could not be sure.

I drove down Princes Freeway towards Geelong, and saw the police checkpoint approaching in the distance. My heart started to race. Get caught trying to fool the police, and I could be apprehended. As I drew nearer to the checkpoint and slowed down, a police officer standing on the side of the road waved at me to stop the vehicle in front of him.

"Hello, sir. Where are you headed today?"

"Hi, I'm going to Geelong. I have work there."

"May I see some proof of your employment there?"

I showed the officer the documents I had brought with me. The officer gave it a quick perusal.

"Thank you, sir, you have a good day."

"Thank you."

As I said the last word, 'you', a sudden burst of excitement choked my throat. I exited the checkpoint but could not get back onto the freeway straightaway. I had to find a spot to stop the car so I could have a heart attack. Immediately after exiting the checkpoint, I saw a side road that led to the countryside. I drove on the rural road for a few minutes until I could not see the checkpoint anymore and stopped the car on the side of the road. As I unclicked the seatbelt and opened the door, I noticed that I was in the middle of an open field. I had arrived at the shire of Golden Plains – a region located halfway between Melbourne and Geelong. The surrounding grass was typical Australian – half green and half yellow. The view was so open in all directions that I could see blobs of cloud become smaller and smaller as they retreated over the far horizon. It was quiet, except for a gentle breeze and the scrunching sound made by the grass as I walked on it. I extended my arms wide and gave a stretch. I felt a gush of freedom run through my body.

After spending a few minutes taking it all in, I took some photos and shared them on my family WhatsApp chat. I got back into the car and continued driving towards my original destination, Ballarat. In the car, I played a YouTube playlist I had prepared earlier, which included 'Take Me Home, Country Roads' by John Denver, and 'I'm Gonna Be' by the Proclaimers. Ballarat, I must say, was underwhelming, mainly because the city was also under a lockdown at the time. Most of the shops were closed. Stores had A4 papers pasted on their doors, some of them with witty messages that made lighthearted mockeries of Dan

Andrews, the incumbent premier of Victoria at the time who had ordered the statewide lockdowns. One of them read, *We'll be back when Dan Andrews says we can*. I made my way to Lake Wendouree, a modest-sized lake in the middle of Ballarat surrounded by some finely maintained horticulture. A lot of Ballaratians were there, either going for a jog or walking the dog. One of the rules in Victoria during the lockdown was that you were allowed to go for one round of exercise per day. Since one round of exercise could mean anywhere from a 5-minute walk to a marathon, people tried to make the most of the rule, taking the opportunity to get out and about and enjoy a daily reprieve from the suffocation of lockdown. I also did one walk around the lake, which took about an hour and a half, and then it was time to head back to Melbourne.

I got home and cooked doenjang-jjigae for dinner – a traditional Korean hot soup made with bean paste and vegetables. The dish was ready just in time when my sister, who I was living with at the time, arrived home from work. Courtney is a pharmacist. Pharmacists, just like other healthcare professionals, had increased workloads during the COVID-19 pandemic mainly because medications suddenly had to be posted to people's homes instead of being picked up at the pharmacy. During the lockdown periods,

Courtney sometimes returned from work and was frustrated because her brother, who was bumming at home all day, did not prepare any dinner. In my defence, I was not in the right state of mind to cook after spending 16 hours a day contemplating the meaninglessness of life. But that day, after my daring daytrip to Ballarat, I felt different and decided that I would show some moral support for a local COVID fighter. The doenjang-jjigae that I made was admittedly not great, but I think Courtney appreciated something hot for dinner.

By the end of 2021, the pandemic had passed its peak. The virus had mutated into a less deadly variant, which allowed the government to carefully direct businesses to reopen. Dental practices across the state had also resumed operations as per normal by mid-late 2021. When the sixth and final lockdown ended on 21 October 2021, Melbourne had become the city with the highest total number of lockdown days in the world. There were six separate lockdowns, spanning over 2 years, with a total of 262 lockdown days. All Melbournians endured a long and gruesome battle. Not everyone survived intact. Many still suffer from the effects of 'long COVID'. The number of mental health conditions soared. I am incredibly lucky that neither my health nor finances were impacted by the pandemic to any complainable degree. I did have to serve two separate courses of 2-week home quarantine, both times because I had come into close contact with an infected person, but the amount of work that I missed out on was nothing compared to millions of Victorians and Australians whose livelihoods were crippled by the pandemic.

I am especially grateful that, in Australia, COVID-19 vaccines were made available across the nation, free of charge, with what I believe to be incredible efficiency. It is a feat that not many countries could pull off during the pandemic. To get a vaccine in Australia, all one had to do was log onto a website, make a booking at a nearby facility, and turn up on the day. Having held a leadership role in the past, I know how difficult it is to set up a system and make it run. I am so proud of all healthcare workers and staff members involved in setting up and running the COVID-19 testing and vaccine facilities across the nation. You guys saved lives.

CHAPTER 10

ON BEING A DENTIST

In December 2021 – 8 years into my dental career – I applied for, and was accepted into, the Bachelor of Arts (BA) degree at Monash University.

During the lockdown periods, I thought about pursuing a study that aligned better with my natural aptitude and talent than dentistry. While I do not regret being a dentist, I unfortunately have to confess – it is not what I am born to do. If I die tomorrow, and my obituary reads that Max was a dentist all his life and nothing more, I will not only turn in my grave but jump back out because I will feel that it has been an inadequate life. This is, of course, not to undervalue those who have dedicated their entire lives in the field of dentistry – I simply feel that my destiny lies elsewhere.

The Bachelor of Arts degree has fascinated me for a long time, because the BA curriculum includes a range of humanities subjects that I have always had a natural appetite for, such as history and philosophy. I could talk about these topics all day, except they are not really considered socially acceptable topics at your everyday gatherings and parties. I remember at a brunch meet-up with friends, I brought up the topic of Immanuel Kant – the father of rationalism – and the table went silent, forcing me to switch the topic. Once, at work, I walked into the sterilisation room and asked a dental assistant, who was busy packaging sterilised instruments, about what she thought of Plato's Theory of Forms. She replied, "Max, I'm working." I had hoped that, by entering a university course, I could meet other like-minded students with whom I could discuss my favourite topics in the world without being dismissed.

The BA degree has been a blast. The contact hours are no more than 10 hours per week, which allows me to maintain part-time work as a dentist. In the lecture rooms, when I am discussing philosophy topics such as the Trolley Problem or Pascal's Wager, or when I am learning about historical topics such as the Cultural Revolution in China or Robespierre's Reign of Terror, I feel that I am in a milieu where my own true self is not only accepted, but celebrated. It is a feeling that I have never experienced while practising dentistry. I am grateful that Monash University has given me a chance to study what I enjoy. By the time this book is published, I will have completed my BA degree. I do not know where the BA degree will take me afterwards. I studied it mainly to satisfy my personal curiosities, not for the purpose of opening up new career pathways. Who knows – if this book sells well and I make millions, I may retire from dentistry and continue being a university student. Let's see how I go.

I am not the only dentist I know who has been exploring alternate pathways outside of dentistry. One dentist I know, who has been an avid badminton player since university days, has set up an online store that sells badminton equipment and wears. Another dentist I know studied MBA and found employment in Germany in a field that is totally unrelated to dentistry. Another dentist went to veterinary school and became a vet. I applaud the decisions made by these guys to make a career switch, and wish that they find meaning and happiness in their new-found pathways.

Those who have switched careers, however, are a minority. Most of my colleagues have stayed faithful to the profession of dentistry. Many have advanced to higher levels of dental studies and become specialists. Those with a more entrepreneurial mindset have opened dental practices and become practice owners. Those with an interest in teaching have successfully organised and convened lectures on dentistry-related subjects. I have no idea how these guys have been able to keep their passion in dentistry alive after so many years. They are the people I am jealous of the most, because they possess a luxury that I do not have – a career that aligns with passion and talent.

Most dentists who graduated with me from Melbourne Dental School are now parents. Half of my Instagram stories are now babies walking around on lawns or in playgrounds. Sometimes they are in the arms of their grandparents. It is heartwarming to see those babies grow and resemble their parents, who are my friends.

In December 2023, I reached an important career milestone – I had been a dentist for 10 full years. A 10-year reunion dinner was held at Melbourne Dental School. I didn't go. I feel that in the age of social media, high school and university reunions are losing their significance. I not only know which brunch café my friends went to last Sunday, but also know exactly what type of coffee they all ordered. I also feel that I already catch up frequently with people that I am close with. Let's be honest – you are not going to make any new best friends at a reunion gathering.

I do not know whether I will still be practising dentistry in another 10 years. They say that you should always think about where you intend to be in 10 years' time and structure your life accordingly. I say, why not stretch that out to 50 years so you can structure a life that works towards your final and ultimate goal? Everyone has different goals in life. Mine is to be able to die smiling. Now, before you laugh at how cringe this sounds, I argue that to be able to smile on your deathbed is more difficult than you imagine. First of all, you cannot be sick, because you cannot smile if the body is in pain. Second, you must have found a sense of fulfilment, so as you depart you can tell yourself that it has been a worthwhile journey. Third, you cannot hold any grudges against other people, because a smile cannot come from a grudging soul. Fourth, there must be peace in your family. You cannot smile if your loved ones are at war with one another. Fifth – and this is probably the most formidable requirement of all – you must overcome the fear of what lies beyond, because one who is in fear cannot smile. Everyone will have different ways of coping with this ultimate fear that all mortals must one day face, such as surrounding oneself with loved ones, or relying on the power of religion. I will have to find my own way. Whether I will still be a dentist in 10 years' time will depend on the extent to which being a dentist can contribute towards my final goal in life, which is to be able to smile on my deathbed.

Being a dentist undoubtedly puts me in a great position to pursue the things I have listed above, such as maintaining a healthy lifestyle and pursuing studies that provide a sense of fulfilment. When I started my BA degree, I cut down my work from 5 days a week to 3 days a week. This is a choice that not many people can afford to make. I imagine that a lot of people would also love to study or pursue things they are passionate about, but have no choice but to give up their dreams and get stuck in a daily grind 5 or 6 days a week because they struggle to make ends meet. Dentistry provides the luxury of free time and disposable income that I can invest in whatever aspect of life I choose. To this end,

I have no right to be anything other than tremendously grateful for the fact that I am a dentist and have a stable job that provides a stable income.

I have been asking myself throughout my career: *Why am I a dentist when there are so many other things I could be?* Being in the dental profession for a bit over a decade has given me an answer: *Sure Max, there are plenty of other things that you could have been, but there is no point mulling over the alternate possibilities when you have been dealt one of the best hands imaginable.* While I maintain that dentistry is not what I am born to do, it does afford me time and money to go on a search for what I *am* born to do. While dentistry is not as lucrative as people make it out to be, it does allow me to lead a comfortable lifestyle and never worry about my personal finances. While the act of fixing teeth does not by itself grant me a sense of fulfilment, being in the dental industry has given me invaluable experiences and life lessons that I will benefit from, for life. And of course, my dental career has produced many stories, some sweet and some bitter, that I can now share with the rest of the dental community by writing this book. If I could go back in time to my high school days and reapply for a university course, would I apply for dental school again? The answer is yes. Ten times out of ten.

Frequently Asked Questions, and Brutally Honest Answers

Q: Doctor, is it going to hurt?
A: Yes.

Q: Doctor, do I need bleaching?
A: No.

Q: Should I brush before or after breakfast?
A: Do you wipe before or after shitting?

Q: Doctor, I brush regularly, so why did I get tooth decay?
A: *Occlusal surfaces*: due to deep fissures. *Palatal/buccal surfaces*: due to deep pits. *Interdental surfaces*: lack of flossing.

Q: Doctor, do I need to replace my silver fillings?
A: Only if it's really necessary.

Q: Doctor, does my son need braces?
A: If he doesn't do it, he'll live. But if he does it, he'll be prettier. It's up to you (or your son).

Q: Doctor, do I need to take out my wisdom teeth?
A: I need to look at your X-ray to answer that.

Q: Doctor, how long will the filling last?
A: It depends on how good my skill is, but I don't want to say that, so I will say instead that it depends on how well you take care of the filling.

Q: Doctor, why is dentistry so expensive?
A: See Chapter 8 of this book – subchapter 'How Much Do/Should Dentists Make?'.

Q: What made you study dentistry?
A: See Chapter 1 of this book.

Q: Does everyone tell you they hate dentists?
A: Only all the time.

Q: Doctor, am I the worst patient ever?
A: Not ever. Just from today.

Q: Should I get an electric toothbrush? Is the normal toothbrush okay?
A: If you're cleaning your room, whether you use a broomstick or a vacuum cleaner, I don't care, as long as you get the job done.

Q: Doctor, can you prescribe me antibiotics?
A: It's best that I don't, but then you'll complain about it to all your friends, so here you go.

Q: Wow doctor, you remember my favourite sport? You have awesome memory!
A: I wrote it in my notes last time so I could pretend that I care.

Q: Doctor, can you prescribe me strong painkillers?
A: Ditto.

Q: Doctor, do I really have to floss every day?
A: No. I only floss once a week (if I remember).

Q: Doctor, who cleans your own teeth?
A: I either do it myself or ask one of my dentist friends to do it for me.

Q: Doctor, you gave me the anaesthetic, but it's still hurting. Why?
A: See Chapter 6 of this book – subchapter 'On Needles'.

Q: Doctor, can I go to the toilet?
A: If you gotta go, you gotta go!

ABOUT THE AUTHOR

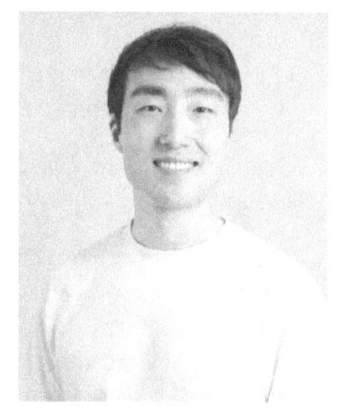

Dr Max Lee is a general dentist who works in Melbourne, Australia. He graduated with a Bachelor of Dental Science degree from Melbourne Dental School in 2013. At his dental clinic, his patients kept asking him why he decided to become a dentist. For the longest time, he could not come up with a suitable answer. One day, Max sat down and wondered, *Seriously, why am I a dentist?* He opened his laptop and started typing. The rest is history.

ENDNOTES

1 Ahpra & National Boards 2023, 'Frequently Asked Questions', viewed 4 October 2024, https://www.ahpra.gov.au/Notifications/Further-information.aspx.

2 Australian Dental Association 2022, *The Australian Schedule of Dental Services and Glossary*, 13th edn, Australian Dental Association, St Leonards, NSW.

3 ChatGPT-4o 2024, *OpenAI*, viewed 29 August 2024. https://chatgpt.com.

4 Australian Taxation Office 2024, 'Tax Rates – Australian Resident', *Australian Government*, viewed 22 November 2024, https://www.ato.gov.au/tax-rates-and-codes/tax-rates-australian-residents.

www.ingramcontent.com/pod-product-compliance
Lightning Source LLC
Chambersburg PA
CBHW022016290426
44109CB00015B/1186